D0672875

MIND BODY DIABETES

TYPE 1 AND TYPE 2

A positive, powerful, and proven solution
to stop diabetes once and for all

Date: 5/30/18

616.462 MAR
Mardlin, Emma,
Mind body diabetes type 1
and type 2 : a positive,

PALM BEACH COUNTY
LIBRARY SYSTEM
3650 SUMMIT BLVD.
WEST PALM BEACH, FL 33406

MIND BODY DIABETES

TYPE 1 AND TYPE 2

A positive, powerful, and proven solution
to stop diabetes once and for all

Emma Mardlin PhD

Clinical Practitioner in Mind Body Medicine

 FINDHORN PRESS

© Emma Mardlin, 2016

The right of Emma Mardlin to be identified as
the author of this work has been asserted by her in accordance
with the Copyright, Designs and Patents Act 1998.

Published in 2016 by Findhorn Press, Scotland

ISBN 978-1-84409-687-9

All rights reserved.

The contents of this book may not be reproduced in any form,
except for short extracts for quotation or review,
without the written permission of the publisher.

A CIP record for this title is available from the British Library.

Edited by Nicky Leach
Cover design by Richard Crookes
Interior design by Damian Keenan
Printed and bound in the EU

DISCLAIMER
The information in this book is given in good faith and is neither
intended to diagnose any physical or mental condition nor to serve
as a substitute for informed medical advice or care.
Please contact your health professional for medical advice and
treatment. Neither author nor publisher can be held liable by any
person for any loss or damage whatsoever which may arise from the
use of this book or any of the information therein.

Published by
Findhorn Press
117-121 High Street,
Forres IV36 1AB,
Scotland, UK

t +44 (0)1309 690582
f +44 (0)131 777 2711
e info@findhornpress.com
www.findhornpress.com

Contents

Dedication

'In loving memory of a major
and inspirational influence on my early life,
My Grandfather, John Savage

and

To my partner Johnny
for being there every step of the way

Acknowledgements

Enormous thanks to Professor Guru Aithal, Dr Stephen Ryder, and Mrs. Andy Mierkalns (Nottingham University Hospitals NHS Trust), for their exceptional array of clinical skills, insight, and continued ability to see the person beyond the patient. Not only did this save my life, it continues to save me from insanity on so many levels!

Everyone with diabetes who has been involved in my research and seen me personally in practice. All your contributions have been courageous and continue to provide invaluable learnings that help us all.

All the inspirational people mentioned throughout this book, whose work continues to change the world and enthuses others to think differently, acknowledging man's infinite capabilities.

A Word From the Author

Over the years, I've experienced phenomenal results from the work and research I've done with diabetes and mind-body medicine – not just individually but with everyone I've worked with. I have more than two decades of personal experience living with Type 1 diabetes myself, so I know all too well what living with this condition entails – a strong sense of humour, a positive attitude, determination, *a lot* of flexibility, and a pretty thick skin. All things you'll undoubtedly relate to.

When it comes to diabetes I've never found too much positivity, encouragement, or pioneering information – whether that's from medical books and physicians, suggested by the media, or found on the internet. As a naturally optimistic person, this drives me crazy on a personal and professional level; there's simply no need for it.

It goes without saying that we need to know the facts, and some people are actually motivated to keep well by all the scary stuff they read. However, I believe this could all be communicated so much better, leading to an exciting and positive way of thinking about diabetes, as alien as that might sound right now.

So, first and foremost, I wrote this book to help you feel a sense of liberation from diabetes as we currently know it. My aim is to shed a completely different light on this condition by sharing new, fresh, and exciting thinking and information. I intend to offer some much-needed positive change, encouragement, and ground-breaking resources within this field to stop diabetes in its tracks – something we can take as far as we choose, which is why it's so exciting. In this book, you'll find no limits about what can be achieved – nothing less than completely lifting the lid on diabetes to break free from this condition!

As with most things, we have to start somewhere, or we'll be stuck in the dark ages of diabetes forever and I, for one, refuse to get stuck anywhere. Life is for living, and this book contains everything to do just that ... to the max. So if you're ready for the same thing – to revolutionize diabetes and break through boundaries – you've definitely picked up the right book. I sincerely hope you get as much value from this book as possible and create some phenomenal, positive changes for yourself. Together, we can create global positive change when it comes to diabetes. So, if you want it, it's all out there. Either way, I'm right with you.

Enjoy your personal journey, and go for it.

Em

A Brief Personal History

In a nutshell, I'm a healthy, fun, determined, independent-thinking individual who loves to embrace life in every possible way – a never-say-never, break-the-boundaries-and-go-for-it kind of person. Professionally, I'm co-founder and partner of The Pinnacle Practice (a health and well-being practice and training company) that I run with my partner of 13-plus years, Johnny. In addition, I write professionally for numerous journals and media.

Even so, my life has been far from a simple stroll in the park, and diabetes has presented me with countless challenges along the way. In fact, if I were to believe just some of the things I've had said to me over the years, I'd probably be off drowning my sorrows in a bar somewhere, with a hospital season ticket in my handbag, and certainly no prospering career. Fortunately, I took no notice and did things my way, or I'd most likely be six feet under by now.

For me, it all began when I was ten years old. I'd been unwell for some time, going back and forth to the doctor's surgery. One evening I was rushed to hospital, severely dehydrated, with excruciating stomach cramps. I was underweight and literally dying of thirst, to the point I finally became unconscious... Well, you know the drill.

I woke up, hooked up to drips and beeping machinery, and saw a nurse sitting by my side. She asked how I was, and for some reason I automatically replied, 'Good, thanks' I think I just figured I wasn't dead, and I felt unbelievably better than before. Well, that or I was still delirious! She then went on to tell me I had something called 'diabetes'.

My reaction was simply to the word: *DI-abetes*. 'Does that mean I'm going to die?' I asked – it was actually something I'd never come across before, so I didn't have a clue. The nurse quickly reassured me, explaining that I could have a completely 'normal' life, but I would have to inject myself daily. She then demonstrated on herself. A medical professional demonstrating what they preach – at the time, I thought that was brilliant!

I think it was my next response that really threw her. 'Is that it? Will I still be able to go on my school holiday to the seaside next week?' I asked.

I'd saved an enormous collection of sweets for this holiday, and needless to say, I was going to be disappointed. I guess I was pushing it by hoping to leave the following week, but I had nothing to lose, so I thought it was worth a go.

Even though I was only ten years old, the fact I was told I wasn't going to die meant that nothing else bothered me. My response from that day on has formed the basis of my philosophy ever since, despite the other challenges I've had to contend with (and there have been plenty). I've never understood why things have to be a problem. There's usually something that can be done to solve a problem or change how we see the situation. In my view, it's a case of taking the lid off the box, having the guts to go for it, and looking at what you *can* do rather than dwelling on what you *can't* change.

Nevertheless, diabetes has tried and tested my belief more times than I care to remember. It's had a nasty habit of creeping up on me when I've least expected it, so I've always had to remain two steps ahead. That can be pretty demanding at times, as you'll know all too well.

I soon learnt that, whatever your situation, when it comes to diabetes, the world doesn't stop and wait, although some people were quick to preach doom and gloom and talk to me about the limitations of diabetes; equally, I found that there were no concessions in life. It's at this point, I felt that there was a pretty clear decision to be made. I could either:

- Never let diabetes stop me, and let the extra determination carry me through, or;
- Surrender to diabetes and get consumed by it. Play the victim, and accept the negative aspersions people can cast (even other people with diabetes, sadly enough) and take everything at face value.

As you can imagine, from the very start, I chose the first option – the one requiring more resilience, tenacity, and courage, but always the more fun, rewarding, and healthy side to be on. But there have been many times throughout my life, when other factors could have easily led me to slip into the second option. I'm not perfect, nor have I had a plain-sailing life.

My first proper sugar low was at primary school the same year I was diagnosed. My teacher had been fully informed about what to look for and how to act in the event that I experienced hypoglycaemia ('a hypo'). Even so, when it did happen, she thought I was acting up, although this was totally out of character for me.

It started when I refused to carry the empty milk bottles. I had no energy, and I began slurring my words, but my teacher didn't realize this was because I was in a low-sugar state and instead, kept me back after school to write lines about not being rude. When I wasn't waiting at the school gate, my mum naturally came looking for me. Immediately realizing I was experiencing a hypo, she intervened and prevented me from lapsing into unconsciousness.

But that's not actually the point.

The following day, the teacher began class by telling everyone about my hypo. Far from an apology being forthcoming, and learning from what had happened (we all make mistakes, right?), she told the class that I was a 'possessed devil' and that I'd been taken over by evil spirits the day before. My classmates looked horrified, and I was so shocked, I didn't know whether to laugh or cry. Instead, I stood up and explained how my sugars had just dropped slightly lower than normal and that I had had a diabetes hypo.

I'd already given the school informative talks about my condition, and how to help if needed, so luckily, my friends and the other kids had more of an appreciation of diabetes than the teacher. I must admit that this still amuses me today, and although I can no doubt be devilish at times, it's certainly not due to my sugar levels dropping.

Things did not improve in secondary school. One teacher insisted on moving me from the top science set to the bottom one, on the grounds that diabetes was making me too tired to cope. I wasn't aware of the reason at the time, and there was no evidence to substantiate such an action, so the move made no sense to me. I pleaded with the lower-set teacher to give me a test, so that I could prove myself and get moved back up again, and fortunately, my results ensured I was. Despite the knocks, persistence paid.

Throughout my schooling (and especially when it came time to think about careers), I came across some pretty limiting beliefs from some figures in authority. I was shocked by how many teachers and other professionals thought diabetes was linked to either being intellectually incapable in some way or equated it with being unable to cope. This always makes me laugh, knowing all the extra things people with diabetes have to manage while, half the time, being more switched on to the world than a lot of people. I was more prepared, more punctual, and got just as good grades as the rest of my classmates, so I put it down to limiting self-beliefs on the part of the staff, based on their own feelings about managing diabetes. Me? I had a life to get on with!

Fortunately, I also had several inspiring teachers – an attitude like that can make the world of difference to an individual. It still amazes me, for example, that after being encouraged by a history teacher, I achieved within the top five percent of students with the highest grade in the country in that year's national exams (and I'm no history genius!). It demonstrates how important support and encouragement are. Even with all the determination or intelligence in the world, positive encouragement makes that extra difference.

Given the work I do now, imagine if I'd become discouraged and given up science? We always accentuate genuine belief, positivity, and support in our practice, because it makes all the difference in how well people feel, respond, and recover.

Despite the lack of encouragement from some quarters, I continued pushing on and entered law school. It was more of a challenge than I had anticipated, though (and that's before I realized law was never going to suit me, anyway). The reason is actually due to some particularly sinister health challenges I was going through from the age of 17 onwards. These were not directly related to diabetes, but they had a huge impact on my condition for quite some time.

I began experiencing a variety of unpleasant daily symptoms. These included low energy and appetite, joint pains, intense dehydration, severe body cramps, nausea accompanied by the vomiting of bile acids several times a day, skin rashes, lack of concentration, intense internal anxiety, odd behavioural changes, suicidal thoughts (that even I knew weren't right), indigestion, a bloated abdomen (I was asked a couple of times when it was due!), and severely inflamed feet, which meant that I was confined to my student halls for a week, thanks to elephant-sized feet. Once, I had so much intense head pain I could barely see, and I lay on the bed for a week, doing everything I could to get it to calm down.

I constantly attempted to find someone who would listen (I'd already called the student GP, but he refused several times to come out). I just wasn't getting anywhere. Eventually, in so much pain, and in a final cry to be heard, I called for an ambulance to get myself admitted to hospital. I just didn't know what was happening to me.

Many of my symptoms were consistent with high glucose levels, but injecting myself caused no improvement; in fact, the amounts I was injecting would have normally sent me dangerously low. Even when I was stabilized in hospital, my symptoms continued. Worst of all was the inability to think clearly. My mind was the one thing I clung to, but over time I felt I was losing that, too. I felt tired, vulnerable, confused, and upset. I even thought I had a brain tumour at one point, and everything was all just some weird illusion. This was so out of character for me.

Even though I was very unwell during this time, I had to endure a great deal of judgement from doctors for not properly managing my diabetes. I continued to protest that something was seriously wrong and it was causing my diabetes to dramatically spiral out of control, and that constantly injecting more and more insulin in an attempt to counteract this resulted in little or no change.

I visited different doctors, trying to make them listen, but of course, I was young and 'that age' and any obscure blood tests were put down to out-of-control diabetes. God forbid anyone should see the person behind the diabetes!

At one point, I was putting on a stone of weight a day due to severe water retention, and sometimes I could hardly recognize myself (actually, I looked like a frog, and it was even worse without makeup). Despite this, I was still told by one GP, 'Sometimes we just have to accept the weight we are, Emma.' He wasn't listening to me. He didn't even check for kidney, liver, or heart dis-ease (it wasn't necessary, apparently). Anyone would think I was a time-waster, eating a tub of salt per day and just needed to stop! But I kept on persisting as I knew my outcome.

This period just before and during university was exceptionally challenging, but I pushed on, made some life-defining decisions, and by remaining focused I got on with the rest of my life.

Since this time, there have been many twists, turns, and curve balls along the way; some of them pretty challenging, too – *but all down to my life events rather than diabetes itself*. These ranged from a coma due to severe hypoglycaemia, being told abruptly I was going blind, and severe gluten intolerance to countless personal challenges and major career developments. All of these I successfully overcame.

Another point here is that whatever else goes on in life, it can affect diabetes, rather than diabetes itself affecting life. In fact 'diabetes' itself has never been the problem, as you'll gather from a host of information and examples that I will share throughout the book.

In successfully overcoming all these experiences, I gained many life learnings, knowledge, and insights from every single aspect along the way. One important thing I will say from all this is that, if the student is aware, willing to learn and respond, the University of Life is the best education any of us will ever get.

After all the lessons I had taken from some quite dramatic events, I ultimately met my life's blueprint in mind-body medicine through exploring psychotherapy further. I had noticed how working with my own mind and having a strong self-awareness directly resulted in positive health improvements physically. I was also increasingly noticing the same improvements with my clients.

More and more, I began to notice the undeniable mind-body link and felt that there was much more to research, explore, and discover on that subject. From a young age, I've often utilized my mind well to control various physical responses, but I knew there was so much more I could learn from the greats within this field and from some of the remarkable case studies I'd come across. I put my energy and focus into studying this, and sometime later, I found my passion in a world of infinite possibility in mind-body medicine.

As a firm believer in practising what I preach, this takes us right back to who I am today: happy, healthy, and well, with a comprehensive and exciting resource and positive support book for you to refer to at any time you wish throughout your own personal journey. Enjoy!

10 Important Pointers Before We Get Going

Before we get into the nitty gritty of this book, there are a few more important things that are good to keep in mind from the beginning.

1. **Am I perfect, and do I know everything?**
   Definitely not, unfortunately! My intention in writing this book is to provide a positive and refreshing perspective on diabetes and experienced support, share some of my personal anecdotes, and above all, provide some good-quality, useful knowledge and resources you can use to get your own great results.

   Whilst I might be an expert in *my own* diabetes and the field of mind-body medicine, please always remember the following:

2. **You are your own expert in your diabetes**
   Your condition is personal to you, so you'll always be the best expert in your own diabetes and needs, as you're the one who lives with it. My intention is to never patronize or preach to you. There's no doubt that there are plenty of volunteers who will gladly do that. That's something that drives me mad, so count me out!

3. **Do I get everything right?**
   No! I'm only human! However, I do learn extremely quickly when things don't go according to plan, and I only focus on what I *can do* to make things right.

   There was actually a challenging time when I was achieving fantastic results with the process of reversing diabetes and then turmoil hit! There were so many emotionally intense things happening in my life at that time, it became extremely tough to focus on my own personal work. At that point I was so disappointed and frustrated, but I soon realized I had to give myself a break and manage what I could, then get back on track when everything settled down. Even though I had to lighten up on my plan, from the groundwork I had previously done there was still a dramatic improvement.

4. **You'll always know best, deep down. Trust yourself.**
   First of all, you'll know when you're ready to take action and make phenomenal changes! If it's not the right time for you, work on what you need to do first (anything holding you back or hinder-

ing you), because if your mind-set isn't in the right place, you'll be working against it, making life hard for yourself. So give yourself a break, and get in the right frame of mind first.

You'll know best when you want support, advice, knowledge, or guidance, or simply when you just want a break and get on with things independently. In either case, you can choose when or what you want to take from this book and make your own decision as to how much value you get from it. Take it or leave it, but it's all there for you when you want it.

5. **Let nothing or no one stop you**
   'Where there's a will, there's a way', and you'll find a lot of resources and personal positive attitude in this book to encourage and support you with that. It is always what *you* believe that really counts and makes the difference as you'll soon discover.

6. **Let it make you rather than break you**
   One of my reasons for writing this book is because I see two choices with diabetes (in any of its forms): it can either *make you* or (all too easily) *break you*.

   That sounds quite dramatic on the face of it, but if you've had diabetes a while, it may resonate with you. Either way, I strongly believe the purpose of diabetes should only ever be to *make you*, and my intention in writing this book is to provide the right resources so it does exactly that. I've had so many experiences where I could have let diabetes nearly break me, but I thankfully recognized this and decided otherwise.

7. **Follow this book**
   If you follow the suggestions in this book and apply the techniques I'm going to share faithfully, you'll dramatically stop diabetes. You will also change your entire outlook on life and achieve your goals. You will never look back!

8. **Life's for living!**
   Let that be your reason for taking positive action. The healthier we are (diabetes or no diabetes), the better, happier, and more fulfilled our lives will be. This then becomes a positive focus, and what we

focus on deep down, we get – happy, healthy, and fulfilled lives! I'll explain this in greater detail later, but it's so important to have a deep-down, positive reason and intention for doing anything. It makes it so much easier to achieve our goals, as we become wholly consistent in our own minds! That goes for anything in life.

9. **Be you – rather than 'a diabetic'! You're so much more than your condition. Never let it define you.**
   One thing you'll notice throughout this book is that I will never re-fer to either you or myself as a 'diabetic'. That is a label that can very easily begin to define a person. No one is a static label – a 'diabetic'. We are so much more than that.

   Refuse to let your health define you. Diabetes is a condition not a person, so never let it hijack you. I always say that no one refers to someone with heart dis-ease as a 'heart attack', or any other perma-nent label. Diabetes, epilepsy, or asthma are no different. *Lose the 'tic', or it will be allowed to 'stick'.*

10. **Think about disease as merely a temporary 'dis-ease'**
    This helps to loosen up what we are programmed to think about 'disease'. It isn't something that has to be static; think of it as a temporary 'dis-ease'. Comfort and ease can be restored when as individuals we're ready to allow this.

Lifting the Lid on Diabetes –
Understanding the Mind-Body Connection

So what has our physical health got to do with our minds? Well the answer to that is ... everything! That is in no way exclusive to diabetes, but those of us with the condition can dramatically benefit from how our minds directly affect us physically.

Here's why.

Although everything I'm about to explain might be completely new information to you, and possibly a lot to digest (generally, because we're not taught this stuff in school), this knowledge has actually been around for some time. Even so, it's often little known, acknowledged, or practised in general medicine, although that is changing.

We're talking about indisputable science – how the human body functions in terms of the health we experience, and how our mind and body interconnect to give us the various physical results we experience every moment of our lives.

I'll explain this in greater detail throughout this chapter, and offer evidence throughout the book, but in a nutshell, this is what you need to know:

Every single thought and emotion we have affects every single cell in our body, because the same electrochemicals that carry our thoughts also bathe every single cell in our body. That's what we mean by the mind-body connection. Our mind and body are constantly communicating with each other in order to function and create our health – mentally and physically (whether we like it or not).

From a scientific point of view, everything we think about affects us physically – from a smile or a frown to health or dis-ease – and as we know, the state of our physical health in turn affects our thoughts and emotions. And so the cycle continues, as shown in the following graphic.

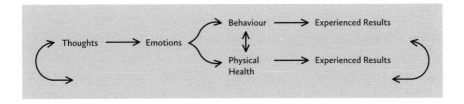

This piece of information is massively exciting. In fact, I would go so far as to say that it's one of the most powerful pieces of information known to man (if properly understood and positively acted upon), as it offers us control over our health and the results we get in life. This is because the way we think, the words we speak, the pictures, sounds, and feelings we hold in our minds are reflected throughout our entire body, and therefore directly affect our physical health.

A Small Practical Exercise You Can Do to Understand How Particular Thoughts Affect Us Physically

First, think of something really funny, such as the last time you nearly lost control laughing. If you're struggling here's one of mine to help.

Rob the Ripper

We were once delivering a business training in a pretty formal setting, and we were yet to break the ice. As we were talking our way through the introduction, one of the most formal-looking people in the room suddenly let off the loudest, longest trump I'd ever heard! And once I start laughing, I can't stop.

Even worse was that no one else in the room flinched, so I couldn't help but think, *Fair enough. Ranging rippers are obviously the norm around here.* Then just as I continued talking in order to distract my-self quickly, the same gentleman got up and popped out of the room pretty sharpish. All we heard were consecutive long, loud rippers (a bit like a moped bike). At this point, I couldn't even look at my partner in case I started laughing. Thank God, someone else finally had a sense of humour and said aloud, 'It's Rob the Ripper' and everyone started laughing. Phew.

Needless to say, poor 'Rob the Ripper' left for that day, so we never saw him again. One of the most natural things in the world can just be so funny in certain situations, and I have to say that was one of them.

Now, as you're hopefully thinking of something funny, try *looking* sad whilst thinking and feeling amused at the same time. Generally, if you really get into the *state* of thinking funny thoughts, you'll find this second part of the exercise nigh on impossible to do. That's because if you're thinking funny thoughts, this tends to automatically be physically reflected as a smile, a laugh, and a good feeling. This is a small but important example of how the way we think affects our emotions and physical state.

On the whole, if you think negatively, you'll feel negative emotions and then display or manifest them physically by either looking flat, crying, being angry, and/or eventually being ill. Basically, a conflicted mind will create conflicted health.

At some point, most of us will have experienced this, such as when we may have been really nervous about something. It will have begun by thinking about the situation in a worried or panicking way, thinking about all the negative 'what if's' (whether this was immediately conscious to us or not); consequently, we'd begin to feel worried, nervous, and anxious. That would then result in us behaving differently (such as forgetting words, having mental blocks and so on). This would then begin to affect us physically, possibly displayed as nausea, shaking, sweating and so on. Then we'd begin thinking about feeling ill, and the negative spiral would continue until eventually a positive distraction breaks the cycle.

But if we think positively to start with, this allows infinite possibilities for exceptional health outcomes; especially where diabetes is concerned.

How?

Well, if we have pleasant, happy, or funny thoughts, this stimulates the release of feel-good chemicals such as *endorphins* for example, and we experience happy feelings, which in turn create optimistic, relaxed, and fun behaviour. Physically, we experience this as a pleasant glow, positive energy, and even pain relief, because endorphins also act as natural painkillers ('endogenous morphine').

The Science Behind This Connection

Such a cycle occurs between the mind and body because all the information that is carried to and within the body is done so in the form of electrical impulses. These electrical impulses are *messages* (information) that are carried from one nerve cell (*neuron*) to the next using an electrochemical called a *neurotransmitter* via one cell communicating with the other, as it transfers this information (a *synapse*).

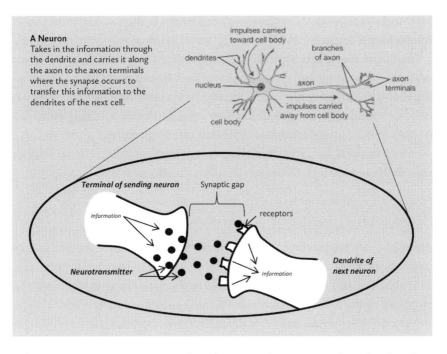

When neurotransmitters were first discovered, scientists thought that they were only found in the brain; in fact, it is now acknowledged that neurotransmitters connect every single neuron in the body, thus forming a network of electrical circuits. Hence, the same electrochemicals that carry our thoughts also carry the very same messages to other cells throughout the body.

Quantum biologists and physicists tell us that neurotransmitters bathe every cell in the human body; therefore, what we think affects every single cell in the body. Effectively, we are constantly sending messages and talking to our bodies. It is this exciting link that brings us to the mind-body connection that makes self-healing, full health, and being free of dis-ease possible. At some point, an unconscious link is formed as to exactly how we will react physically to our thoughts and emotions; hence we manifest dis-ease, illness, and conditions differently. This physical manifestation has metaphorical significance when we take the time to analyze this link.

Energy and Emotions

Through the mind-body connection, our emotions (instigated by our thoughts and all that we hold in our minds) become a form of energy, and when this energy is negative, it manifests in the body as dis-ease or illness.

The negative message is sent to every cell in the body, causing us to physically reflect a negative health state.

In this respect, bad backs can often be an example of being weighed down by something and reflect that we don't have a particular support in life that we're looking for – emotionally, financially, or in whatever way is relevant. Similarly, stomach ulcers may reflect something eating away at a person. Shoulder problems may represent carrying a burden in life.

More importantly, we can change this at any point in order to achieve full health and healing; in this case, to stop diabetes.

How Is It Possible For Us To Change Our Health Once Our Cells Have Already Been Affected In a Particular Way?

All our cells have intelligence and memory. It is widely reported that 98 percent of atoms in the body are different from what they were a year ago, as confirmed and clearly explained by Dr. Deepak Chopra, although the structure of the bone cells may remain fairly constant:

- The skin is new every month;
- The stomach lining is new every four days;
- The liver is new every six weeks;
- Our red blood cells are new every three months;
- We are therefore constantly changing.

As a pioneer within mind body medicine, Dr. Chopra highlights how science has even proved that damaged nerve cells can actually sprout new growth (Deepak Chopra, 1989[1]). From such information, we see how the body has infinite healing possibilities. We can liken the body in this way to the water cycle; a constant flow of new water, ever changing throughout its journey, hence you never get wet by the same rain. This also highlights how change is naturally a sign of life. Change is what allows us to positively move forward and progress. Change within the body is no different.

So Why Do We Still Look the Same and Hold Onto Dis-ease? What Is Cell Memory?

The only reason we still look, sound, and feel the same and hold onto disease, illness, or chronic conditions is because we have 'cell memory': our cells remember what to do – good and bad. We already know that organ donors can pass on character traits and memory through their organs, and that cellular memory can be inherited, as well as the notion of muscle memory, so we know that our cells hold memory.

Supporting this notion of cell memory is a particular experiment conducted by a French immunologist, Dr. Benveniste[2]. He created what was effectively 'a bad allergy' in a test tube. When pushing the boundaries of this experiment by reaching the point of only adding water rather than the original trigger used and needed to evoke the reaction, he found the reaction was still set off with the same power as before.

This experiment therefore found that you can trigger the immune system without anything actually (physically) being present! Basically, the same reaction as before occurred completely from memory. Human white blood cells still acted as if they were being attacked, leaving cellular memory as the main plausible answer. So when it comes to the mind-body, unless we can learn from our memories and release any linked negative emotions that are held as negative cell memory, we are likely to incubate the memory of dis-ease and experience its effects continually.

What is interesting is that this memory isn't just of cell functionality but of emotional memory, too, and it is the emotional memory that consequently alters the functionality. This is pertinent to diabetes and any chronic (long-term) conditions – the cells are remembering to malfunction, and must rely on external intervention (injecting or medicating) in order to function effectively.

In considering the concept of memory, scientific studies showed that after rats had been trained to run a maze and then had nearly all their brain tissue removed, they still remembered how to run the maze, albeit a little slower (Karl Lashley 1929, 1950[3]). This led neuroscientist Karl H. Pribram[4] to postulate that memories were not stored in a single neuron or exact location in the brain, but were spread over the entirety of a neural network; effectively memory is stored holographically, sporadically throughout our entire body (and brain). Again, this emphasizes the undeniable mind-body connection and its significance.

It is therefore vital to fully resolve any negative emotions attached to memories, rather than storing them within the body. If we continue to transmit negative messages throughout our nervous system in this way, they will only manifest physically as dis-ease.

The exciting news is that when cell memory is not ideal or healthy, we can reprogramme it by releasing stored negative emotion and using guided visualization, as well as many other techniques to retrain the functionality of the cells. Such processes and techniques will be discussed in detail later. They are resources you can use to experience positive changes, and that will inevitably lead to phenomenal results in stopping diabetes.

In releasing stored negative emotions we can then get the positive and productive, healthy results we want. It's probably also worth mentioning here that the longer our cells have learnt to do something, the longer they may take to retrain. Everything is a process, a positive step towards our end goal, so keep taking action, keep positive, and keep focused.

> As part of my own personal research in this field, I addressed and released many different negative emotions and traumas that had manifested throughout my past (some very severe to me and some not at all), as well as applying other techniques. As a result, I witnessed some amazing results. My health consistently and dramatically improved to the point that I only required 16 units of insulin per day with a HbA1C of 5.7 percent (approx. average of 6.7 mmol/l and 120 Mg/dl) and eating a regular, balanced diet.
>
> Then emotional disruption hit – in a pretty big way, too – and I was sent off course! I was aware of the effects of this, and I had the resources to manage it very well, but just to give you some idea of the impact of negative emotion on health, I suddenly required 40 units of insulin/ day, had a HbA1C of 7 percent (8.5 mmol/l & 154 Mg/dl), and I wasn't eating any more or less in comparison to before.
>
> This shows how negative emotion could have knocked me off course far worse, had I not known how to manage this.

There are many fascinating examples of how the mind-body connection has had some amazing results in terms of full health and healing, as well as how it causes ill health in the first place. Remember: The thoughts, pictures, sounds, and emotions we hold in our mind dramatically affect our physical health.

The physical mind and body interconnection is shown in the diagram on the following page.

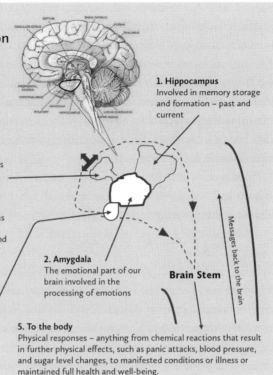

The Physical Mind-Body Communication Loop

(From *The Brain to the Body*)

1. Hippocampus
Involved in memory storage and formation – past and current

2. Amygdala
The emotional part of our brain involved in the processing of emotions

Brain Stem

Messages back to the brain

3. Hypothalamus
Orders physiological responses to emotions – often through hormones that may stimulate a positive, survival, or negative physical response, such as 'corticotrophin', which then causes the pituitary to release a further hormone that causes the adrenal glands to release the stress hormone 'cortisol'. This results in the physical responses we know as 'stress'. The physical effects induced by this process in the mind will be discussed in the following pages, so you can directly see the mind body connection.

4. Pituitary gland
produces further Hormones that control other glands, resulting in physical responses.

5. To the body
Physical responses – anything from chemical reactions that result in further physical effects, such as panic attacks, blood pressure, and sugar level changes, to manifested conditions or illness or maintained full health and well-being.

In a Nutshell

The *amygdala* shown in the illustration plays a large part in the emotional stimulus, because this brain structure relays information among the other brain regions, including the *hippocampus,* which is involved in memory, and the *hypothalamus*, which stimulates hormones and other chemicals in response to specific emotions. This includes those derived from our experiences, as well as those related to stored and current memories from everything we think and choose to take in through our senses.

These hormones and chemicals are responsible for further changes (often via the pituitary and thyroid gland) that result in the physical responses we experience. As noted earlier, if we think something is good, for example, we feel happy and the brain releases endorphins (feel-good brain chemicals), which in turn cause the physical response of wellness and lower the ability to feel pain. This loop continues, as affected organs 'report and send back signals' by electrochemical impulses to the brain. That, in turn, causes further emotional and physical responses to take place. This is the mind-body connection in terms of how we all experience health. This physical mind-body connection therefore highlights an entire network of information, whereby the mind and body become one and the same as a result of neurochemicals. Excitingly this is so much so that insulin has been found to exist and function in the brain.[5] Irrespective of whether insulin is of peripheral origin or actually produced in the brain, insulin is suggested to act through its own receptors present in the brain. This leaves us with endless opportunities as to what we can achieve with a mind-body diabetes approach.

It may also explain why I have noted a significant difference in blood sugar results (all other factors being equal) when I apply a specific visualization technique, compared with when I don't.

The Relevance of the Mind-Body Connection Specifically Related to Diabetes and Stress

When we feel stress, the hypothalamus secretes a hormone called *corticotrophin releasing factor* (CRF), which mediates the release of *adrenocorticotrophic hormone* (ACT) from the pituitary gland. That, in turn, directs the adrenal cortex to release the stress hormone *cortisol* into the bloodstream. Cortisol is a potent immune system suppressor that also elevates blood pressure and blood sugar. Both cortisol and *adrenaline*, another stress hormone, cause the liver to break down stored glucose (*glycogen*) and release it into the bloodstream as *glucose*, amongst many other undesirable responses associated with stress, such as racing heartbeat. This therefore can create a negative spiral when you are managing diabetes.

The process above is referred to as the *HPA (hypothalamic-pituitary-adrenal) Axis*. As well as helping you to control your reaction to stress, trauma, and injury, it importantly also helps to control temperature, blood pressure, digestion, the immune system, mood, sexuality, and energy use. This is why when we allow ourselves to become stressed and this interconnected system becomes out of balance, we physically experience such effects.

In my own case, I've seen how intense periods of stress have resulted in elevated sugar levels, which have then resulted in the need for additional insulin. That in turn creates other challenges.

Therefore, in direct relation to the mind and body, unless we can learn from our negative memories and any subsequent negative thoughts and emotions linked to them, we are likely to incubate the memory of dis-ease and experience its negative effects continually.

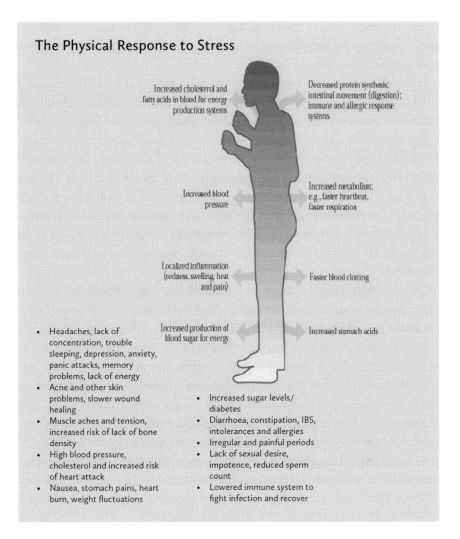

The Physical Response to Stress

Increased cholesterol and fatty acids in blood for energy production systems

Decreased protein synthesis; intestinal movement (digestion); immune and allergic response systems

Increased blood pressure

Increased metabolism; e.g., faster heartbeat, faster respiration

Localized inflammation (redness, swelling, heat and pain)

Faster blood clotting

Increased production of blood sugar for energy

Increased stomach acids

- Headaches, lack of concentration, trouble sleeping, depression, anxiety, panic attacks, memory problems, lack of energy
- Acne and other skin problems, slower wound healing
- Muscle aches and tension, increased risk of lack of bone density
- High blood pressure, cholesterol and increased risk of heart attack
- Nausea, stomach pains, heart burn, weight fluctuations

- Increased sugar levels/ diabetes
- Diarrhoea, constipation, IBS, intolerances and allergies
- Irregular and painful periods
- Lack of sexual desire, impotence, reduced sperm count
- Lowered immune system to fight infection and recover

Common Colds and Flu – Why We Never Need to Be in the 'Vulnerable' Group

Many people think we get colds as a result of a change in the weather, automatically passing it on, going outside with wet hair, or even worse, because people (like those with diabetes) are classified in a 'vulnerable' group. Interestingly, colds originate from none of these factors.

Some of the above-mentioned scenarios can certainly worsen a cold or make an individual more susceptible to catching one, but colds and flu are actually triggered when we are overrun, strained, and become emotionally run down or experience some form of emotional congestion. This leads to

stress, tiredness, and a weakened immune system, making us more susceptible to germs and viruses (like rhinopharyngitis) that then manifest as a
cold or flu.

It's no coincidence the cold and flu season occurs in winter, around
the holiday season. Christmas isn't called 'the silly season' for nothing; it's
fuelled by emotion for one reason and another – from parties and overin-
dulging to family gatherings! At this time of year, we all tend to rush around
in preparation for the 'big day', setting us up for colds. In addition to this,
is the constant focus on colds in the media, from relentless cold and flu advertising, flu jab circulars and promotions, to general advertising portraying
colds during the winter months. This almost primes us to get sick. Is it any
wonder so many people get colds when our neurology is surrounded by so
many suggestions of getting one? It's actually beginning to sound like mass
'negative' hypnosis.

Again this is a great example of the mind-body connection, because we
are generally programmed to think we can 'catch' a cold, or that we're expected to get one; we willingly oblige.

If you want more evidence that it takes a lot more than a virus for us
to catch a cold, there are numerous scientific abstracts linking stress and
the common cold that you can read.[6] It is also known how experimenters
once incubated cold viruses, placed them directly on the mucous lining of
the noses of volunteers, and found that only 12 percent of the subjects ever
came down with a cold. Even further tests, which exposed subjects to drafts,
cold water, and other external environmental factors, did not increase this
percentage.[7] This quite dramatically highlights that it's not actually the case
that we necessarily catch a cold; it's more about what we think, what we
expect, and how our emotions manifest physically.

Colds are yet another example of a particular mind-set escalating to the
point of manifesting physically in the body. This is why the way we think is
so imperative to our health!

Always of this belief, I've never had my 'priority/ vulnerable group' flu jab
for more than 18 years, and I've also never had the flu, either. On the rare
occasion I have had a cold, each and every time I've known exactly why –
I've been run down and the cold has been a physical expression of my emotional state. Any colds I've had have passed very quickly; in fact, I've worked
some intense 18-hour days during colds, and they have never stopped me.
So there's a lot to be said for emotional well-being and awareness of our
internal emotional state in managing our overall physical health.

Really Lifting the Lid on Diabetes and Thinking Differently

When I talk about 'lifting the lid' on diabetes, I'm referring to the unexpected results we can achieve by working to positively influence our minds. Incredibly, we can do this by using a series of techniques, resources, and above all the right mind-set. This will enable us to really utilize the power that is deep within our minds to stop diabetes forever, an exciting prospect. We often hear it said that we only use approximately ten percent of our mind. This means that we have so much more capacity to unleash to get truly phenomenal results.

A huge and little-understood part of the mind tends to run on autopilot, maintaining the entire nervous system without us having to constantly think about it. For example, while you have been sitting here reading, and perhaps drinking a nice cup of tea or coffee, you have no doubt been unaware of having to breathe in and out constantly in order to stay alive, or the feeling of the floor beneath your feet, or your pulse rate, or your temperature regulation (or at least not all of them at once, because you'd be exceptionally distracted if you did). But it is this part of your mind that is running the *autonomic nervous system* (involuntary activity) and your entire body without you having to consciously think about it. It is doing vital work to keep us alive that is most often out of our awareness.

This part of the mind also stores all our experiences – past, present, and future, it's all in there. This is why it's possible to only recall certain memories at certain times, because it would be very challenging to think about all these memories and experiences all at once.

Amongst many other amazing attributes, this part of the mind represses negative memories with negative emotions; however, it will intermittently present these memories for resolution (a bit like tapping you on the shoulder every so often). When negative memories and experiences are left unresolved, negative emotions begin to manifest. This is when this wonderful part of the mind is interrupted from running, maintaining, and preserving the body to the blueprint of perfect health for which it was originally designed. This is how we begin to manifest illness, dis-ease, and various conditions that develop over time.

It's important to let go of and fully resolve any negative emotions, trauma, and experiences, so that we have an opportunity to manifest the best possible health and healing. We can learn how to tap into this powerful part of the mind to get the maximum results to dramatically improve diabetes and overall health. This book focuses on how we can use this amazing and often undiscovered part of our minds to dramatically change and improve our health.

One last thing before we get started. This part of our mind should never be underestimated. It is truly the biggest asset and resource we have. If we respect it and look after it (as if it is our own child in our care), we will be respecting and looking after ourselves in the best way we can to achieve optimal health and well-being.

I'll refer to this part of the mind as the 'unconscious', because it is out of our awareness until it becomes 'subconscious'. Through being aware that the unconscious exists and that there may be unresolved things we need to attend to, we will know to look out for any signals it may be sending us that are prompting us to take action. This often manifests as ill health in varying degrees.

For example, if I were to suddenly start getting bad colds, it would be a sign that I need to look at why I am getting burdened and run down. What really is the problem? It might be not having the right balance in life by being overloaded with work. It might be not paying myself enough attention. There are many possible reasons. Either way, a bad cold reflects my unconscious mind not running my body properly and giving me a prompt to look at something deeper that I need to address in order to restore my health. It's through having this awareness and using the tools to do something about it that will always bring about amazing health and well-being.

CHAPTER ONE SUMMARY

- Every single thought and emotion we have affects every single cell in our body because the same electrochemicals that carry our thoughts also bathe every cell throughout the body. That's the mind-body connection. Our mind and body are constantly communicating with each other (whether we like it or not).
- Our thoughts affect our emotions, and these directly affect our physical health and behaviour (from a sniffle to chronic conditions).
- Getting stressed causes a hormone release that has dramatic negative physical effects.
- Our physical health is metaphorical of our thoughts and emotions.
- We can effectively work with our minds to activate and restore positive health.
- Our bodies are constantly changing. We only hold onto dis-ease because our cells store memories and remember what to do.

- We can release negative emotion attached to memories and retrain our cells.
- The mind has infinite capabilities to achieve health, healing, and well-being.

The Question Set –
A Good Starting Point

The question set described in this chapter is a great starting point to help you make certain discoveries that can lead to amazing results and future health comparisons.

It's quite thought-provoking, and a good personal indicator of our current health results and how we might currently feel about things. In addition, it's a concrete way of assessing our experiences and linking them to our thoughts and emotions and overall health.

When you answer the questions and see this information in black and white, it may look different or even surprise you, because you'll be able to gauge certain patterns that otherwise wouldn't be obvious. These patterns will be most apparent if you read the answers to the questions out loud. Answering these questions will allow you to highlight essential patterns and work out what you need to do to positively change and release certain key areas in your life, and it will make a huge difference to your results.

If you answer these questions honestly, with an open mind, you'll quickly become aware of what you need to work with in both your mind and body, using the resources and information throughout this book.

It's good to revisit this questionnaire once you've applied all the techniques and processes in this book and worked on any areas you initially picked up on. This allows you to compare for yourself how much you experience things differently and is guaranteed to get you on the path to phenomenal results, when applied thoroughly.

I have compiled this question set myself and also use it for my own health. I've been surprised by how many times I've initially missed things and, indeed, continue to realize certain points every time I do this exercise. So writing it down or talking it through really helps to identify where you might want to start, as you may not necessarily realize any of these patterns consciously or before you begin.

I've put all of the questions below so you can answer them on a separate sheet and use them as many times as you like. I've also added a guide to what each question means and how the answer will specifically help. Based on my own experiences using this question set, I know just how thought-provoking and powerful these questions can be as a baseline to work from.

A Few Pointers About the Questions

There are no right or wrong answers; we're all individuals and manage things differently. So be honest; it's just a guideline for going forward. The idea is that whatever the answers are to begin with, you can change the outcome to one you prefer.

- Avoid feeling disappointed or that you *should* be writing something else. The more information you can give, the better the results. Remember who you're doing this for.
- Because this work is for you, it's about what *you* think. Some things may be tough to admit and confront, but this is for your benefit alone, no one else's. Keep focused on that and your highest intention for doing this work in mind.
- Some questions may seem a little obscure, but they are included here for a logical reason. They will definitely make sense when we start the work towards the intended outcome, I promise!
- Please reject any questions you find irrelevant or have no meaning to you.
- Be sure to note the date when you complete your first question set, so that you can gauge your progress and measure your successful changes when you next do it.

The Questions

1. How long have you been diagnosed as having diabetes?
2. Is your diabetes T1 or T2?
3. When is the last time you were admitted to hospital related to diabetes?
4. What is your current medication regime (type and dosage/duration)?
5. What was your last HbA1c or roughly your average blood sugar taken?
6. What is your current diet, lifestyle, and exercise regime?
7. Do you ever feel labelled as a 'diabetic', or do you even label yourself?

8. What are your general thoughts, opinions, views, and feelings about having diabetes?
9. What do you find is personally the most challenging aspect of having diabetes?
10. Are there any points about having the condition that you actually like or wouldn't want to let go of? *For example, special attention, privileges, perks and so on.*
11. How old were you when you were diagnosed?
12. What was the most challenging part you found about diagnosis?
13. Do you experience any complications of the condition?
14. Do you have any specific allergies/intolerances? *For example, milk or gluten.*
15. Do you have any other conditions (also any not necessarily related to diabetes)?
16. At your time of diagnosis, or even several years prior to this, did you experience any traumatic events, shock, loss or bereavements, or any form of negative emotion or experience?
17. In your opinion, what is the real root cause of your diabetes (the emotional root)? *Write the first thing that comes to mind, no matter what this may be.*
18. Have you ever experienced depression or low mood as a consequence of diabetes? How and why? What was the root of this?
19. Have you ever experienced significant depression before having diabetes? How and why? What was the root of this?

** Please strongly reject this next question if it does not apply **

20. Have you ever used diabetes to self-harm? For example, overeating, undereating, not injecting, punishing yourself in some way, and so forth? If so, why was this? Keep asking yourself the question 'For what purpose?' and note it down.
21. What emotion or emotions would you connect with having diabetes, or if diabetes was an emotion what might it be? *For example, sadness, fear, guilt, and so on.*
22. Do you see or feel your diabetes is a part of you or that it is you?
23. Do you ever feel your management of diabetes is being judged by professionals, or do you ever feel a pressure from others to have perfect control? Does this bother you?

24. Do you feel you have a good support network, such as family, friends, and medics? How could this be improved to best help you? What can you do to help change this? What needs explaining, can you talk openly to them? Are you around the right supportive and encouraging people to best help you?
25. If you could change one thing about having diabetes, what would it be and for what purpose?
26. If you could change anything about the way diabetes is treated what would it be? What can you do to help achieve this?
27. Does your condition dramatically impact upon your daily life or prevent you from doing anything you'd like to do?
28. What is your ultimate purpose and goal for reading this book? What is your specific outcome that you would like to happen?

Congratulations! I know it can seem long-winded, but this information can help to make great changes. I appreciate some of the questions may not always make immediate sense, but as we progress through the book, they soon will. By using these results we can now work out what really needs to happen to dramatically improve and stop diabetes for you personally.

Working Through the Results

As you read through these explanations, take a highlighter carefully back through your answers, and highlight any prominent words, re-occurring factors, negative emotions, or 'life limitations' – a life limitation refers to anything you think or believe that stops you from getting what you want. This will help you to get real solutions and results in using this book, particularly how to make good use of Chapters Five and Six. You'll also notice a huge difference after you complete this work, when you revisit the question set and have totally different answers!

The following are some notes on each of the questions as a guideline to help you as you go through your answers.

Question One

A longer diagnosis can sometimes (though not necessarily) mean that it will take a little longer to dramatically improve your health and for the body to readjust than a shorter diagnosis length. This is simply because the body has had longer to adjust to diabetes, so it's just a case of needing to train a little more than a newly diagnosed person. This also has a lot to do with the natural remaining beta cell function at the point of diagnosis, too. A longer diagnosis can potentially indicate a lot more things to think about and work on because they will have had a longer time to accumulate and manifest. This is a bit like washing an old stain – it takes a bit longer to get it out than a fresh surface stain. This is perfectly natural, and you'll get just the same great results; however, it's important to note that on occasion, you might need to be a little more patient in allowing time for things to resolve. I'm talking from experience. In the grand scale of life, even a couple of years to fully see a dramatic change or completely stop diabetes isn't long in comparison to a lifetime with the condition.

Question Two

In long-term T1 diabetes, there will be more retraining of the body to do in order to readjust, simply because at least 70 percent of beta cells will have been destroyed within the first three years of diagnosis, and most if not all of them any time after.[8] In T2 diabetes, it will be easier to more quickly retrain the body and readjust. Studies have shown that with the right commitment, this has been done in as little as eight weeks with specific diet and lifestyle changes (see Chapter Six for details).

Questions Three, Four, Five, and Six

Provides a great comparison to see and track your progress before, midterm, and so on, until you reach your specific goal. Avoiding any hospital admissions is a good indicator of great management and significant wellbeing. Tracking your medication dosage and type will indicate major changes and progress alongside improved HbA1c results. Seeing current diet, lifestyle, and exercise regimes in black and white can help you to see where you can make new adjustments in this area of your life (especially after reading Chapter Six).

NOTE: The best pattern is a decrease in insulin or medication, with a decrease in HbA1C and daily blood glucose levels, whilst maintaining a regular healthy lifestyle.

Question Seven

This question just brings about an awareness of how you feel with regard to being labelled, and even whether you label yourself. If this is highlighted, then adopting the mind-set talked about in this book will help with this, so that you can discover who *you* really are, diabetes aside. Remember: What you believe and focus on, you get and become. This may also highlight any limiting beliefs (certain beliefs that can limit you from fully achieving everything you are capable of) that need to be addressed using the resources in Chapter Five.

Question Eight

This is a chance to 'blow out' your thoughts. Having done this you can highlight any negative emotions and limitations and realize what your general focus is. Is this positive and looking towards what you want? Or is it more negative, looking in the direction of what you want to avoid?

A Personal Example

In my first answer to this question, I noted the word 'inconvenience' cropping up a few times. So I asked myself *Why is it an inconvenience?* I arrived at tiredness when working, regular toilet trips, nausea, and so forth. *Why is that a problem?* Because I feel ill and find it hard to concentrate when working. *Why do I feel so tired and ill?* High sugar levels. *Why do I have high sugar levels?* I've been neglecting myself and putting everything and everyone else first. *Why do I feel the need to do this?* If I focus on myself I feel depressed. *For what purpose and why do I feel that depressed that I need to reflect this through diabetes?* Now I arrive at the root cause of this problem, and I can work out what I really need to work on in order to fully resolve the problem.

So you can see how this will lead to the very core emotional problem that can then be highlighted as something to work on and release later, all just from picking up on the words you use without even thinking about it. It's a good way to become aware of how your language can reflect how you might be really feeling about something.

Question Nine

This helps to highlight any current worries or concerns that can be later worked on and resolved throughout.

Question Ten

This is important because it refers to something we call 'secondary purpose'. Believe it or not, this simply means when a person has a motive as to why they would want to hold onto a condition.

A common secondary purpose, or gain, may occur as a result of the illness itself and the 'attention' the sick person receives from a loved one who acts more caring and devoted towards them as a result of their illness. In this type of situation, recovery takes longer because the person gains in another way from being ill.

In the case of secondary gain, it's always important to look at the highest intention in that person's life; that is, the purpose behind someone benefiting from a seemingly negative situation. In the example cited above, the person's highest intention is to be loved in order to live a happy and fulfilled life, but they feel that they can only meet this need when they are ill.

Especially in the case of diabetes (but generally, too), if a person doesn't look after themselves, their highest intention to be happy and live a fulfilled life will be seriously limited, anyway, so in this respect secondary gain doesn't actually serve any positive purpose. On the other hand, if the person gets well, they can find another way to seek the love they were initially seeking – by addressing the real problem of why they feel they aren't getting enough ordinarily. They can then live a fulfilled life, which is actually the same intention as the secondary gain, so we may as well release any secondary gains and find more positive ways to achieve the same thing.

Secondary Gains

I once saw a client who had done exceptionally well to conquer a very serious mental health condition, and they were very nearly off all their medication and had reduced all the nasty side effects. This meant they were finally ready to fully take the plunge and let go of this condition; however, my client actually said to me that whilst they knew they could do this, they felt that they couldn't, because the specific financial state benefits they got for this condition really helped them and they weren't prepared to manage without these particular benefits. In this case, the gain of the benefits outwon the full release of their condition due to the 'secondary gain'. A secondary gain is a big limitation and needs to be removed first.

Question Eleven

The age of diagnosis can help to work out anything that may have been happening around that time to cause you excess stress or negative emotion. It also helps to work out how you might have been influenced at that time, such as finding the root of any limitations you feel about diabetes currently.

For example, certain beliefs can stick with us and influence our thinking, even more so when we are children.

As I wrote earlier, when I was newly diagnosed, my parents were great, and we got on with things in a positive way; however, my teacher (the one who called me a 'possessed devil' during my first hypo in class) was another matter. I could have let her influence me into thinking that diabetes is something to be ashamed of, but luckily, I didn't care, and I was able to get on with my life without being negatively influenced by her.

Answering this question allows you to highlight any patterns or issues that need to be recognized, worked on, and changed if you have any deep-rooted negative beliefs and limitations about diabetes. It all comes from somewhere.

Release Limiting Beliefs

One of my clients confided in me that he thought there was nothing he could do about his Type 2 diabetes, and he was feeling very depressed and defeated. When I asked him what led him to conclude that this was the case, he explained that his GP had told him at diagnosis, 'Once a diabetic, you'll always be a diabetic. There's nothing you can do about it, so just get on with it.' Well, after being told that, how would this poor guy imagine anything else, I thought! But as soon as he released this limiting belief through our work, he learnt otherwise. The difference in him was phenomenal. Needless to say, he changed his GP and has never looked back.

Question Twelve

Noting the most challenging thing about your diagnosis will allow you to see if this is something that has gone, because you've already addressed it, or whether it is something more prevalent that has stuck with you and needs currently addressing in order to let it go.

If it's a case of the latter, note it down and get to the root of this, in order to work on it later. When you work with these questions again, it will be interesting to see if the problem is no longer there.

Question Thirteen to Question Fifteen

These questions highlight any other areas you might need to work on first. This is because it can be best to address any complications or other potential health conditions / allergies that may prevent you working on healing your diabetes. In that case, you can still use all the resources in this book and apply them to all other areas, too.

It's also important to work out what the emotional root cause of your complication is, so you can improve or stop it. This is also useful for when you answer the question set again, so that you can track your progress and improvements overall.

Important Note Regarding Complications

When diabetes control undergoes a rapid and significant improvement, complications associated with the condition *may* slightly worsen in the short term – but dramatically improve in the long term. It is important to take things slowly. For example, work on each issue one step at a time, addressing and stabilizing any complications first, and always treat this as a positive ongoing process, to avoid any slight disappointments if you do experience a setback on other fronts. This is not written in stone, but it's best to stay mindful of the potential for this happening. Be sure to keep your focus positive, so as not to expect or anticipate this and create a self-fulfilling prophecy. It's not always the case!

Question Sixteen

This is one of the most important questions because it helps you find the emotional root cause of your diabetes. When you realize and release it, you'll experience the most significant changes in your work. This requires complete honesty, though, and digging until you get to the real root cause.

Question Seventeen

This is important because it is about what you *think* is the emotional root cause. It's important to make a note of it, so you can work to release it. Doing so will help bring about a dramatic improvement in your diabetes, as it will bring to light the mind-body connection involved and the negative emotion that manifested physically as diabetes.

Question Eighteen

This relates to experiencing depression as a consequence of diabetes, in order to highlight any more negative emotion or limitations that need recognizing and releasing. This can also help to highlight a motivation to dramatically improve diabetes in order to let go of a nasty debilitating challenge like depression.

Question Nineteen

If you experienced depression before diabetes, answering this question may well help to uncover more emotional root causes (sometimes more prevalent with T2 diabetes but not exclusively). Keep digging. Ask yourself, *For what purpose was I depressed?* When you get to the real emotional root, make a note of it and recognize it as a big one to release.

Question Twenty

If you have used your diabetes diagnosis as a reason to self-harm (which, unfortunately, isn't uncommon, probably because it can be so easy to do), keep asking yourself *Why?* Until you get to the emotional root cause of this – *For what purpose am I doing this?*

Become aware of the negative actions you have been taking, and know that you have the power to **STOP** them immediately and do something about them by understanding yourself and your need – *What has to happen in order for me to stop this now?* Really keep going with this question, then release the core negative emotion linked to it, using the resources in Chapter Five.

Question Twenty-One

These particular emotions are important because they can highlight root causes. It is necessary to recognize any negative emotions that you link with your condition, in order to release them.

Even if you have highlighted positive emotions in connection with your diabetes, ask yourself if these are just a positive take on something not so great – or could they be a reason you might want to hang onto diabetes? This takes honesty and reflection on your part, as positive emotions are relevant, too.

Question Twenty-Two

Although this question may seem a little odd, it's actually very important because it allows us to recognize how we see diabetes. If you see your diabetes and yourself as a person as being one and the same, it may well mean you've let diabetes consume you or have become identified with it, and feel reluctant to let it go.

If this is the case, you need to ask yourself who you are as a person without diabetes: *What purpose does diabetes really serve for me? Is it making up for another need that really needs fulfilling?*

If you don't know how to answer those questions, think about who you really want to be? Release the real inner you. Going through the Guided Goals and Outcomes section in Chapter Nine in detail will help you answer this. It may also be necessary to release the negative emotion of *fear* in order to do this, if something is holding you back. For more on this, refer to Chapter Five.

If you feel that diabetes is 'a part of you', is it a part you need? What does that part represent? What purpose does it serve? And what emotionally has to happen in order for you to let it go? Make a note of all your answers and any specific work you might need to do in order to help yourself address and overcome this.

Question Twenty-Three

This question relates to any external pressures you might be feeling. If this is the case, they can cause undue stress and distract from a positive focus on what's really important. It will help to read the section on Judgement in Chapter Five.

Question Twenty-Four

This question is about whether you feel you have a good support around you. If you do, this will always make improving diabetes much easier. Generally, the people around us and the environment we're in can influence us dramatically, whether we realize it or not, so it's important to be around positive, supportive, and encouraging people as much as possible – it just rubs off! Unfortunately, negativity breeds like wildfire.

If you don't have a good support network, work out what you can do to change this, and communicate your feelings in different ways. You will find a lot of resources throughout this book covering how to do this. Our support network and the people we are around are so important in terms of who we are, who we become, and what we can achieve. Which is why, you always have a positive support here.

Accentuate the Positive

I once met a young girl who was newly diagnosed with diabetes. Her parents introduced me to her in order to give her some encouragement because she was really struggling with things. After talking to her for a while, I discovered that she had picked up some really negative and daunting things from an online diabetes forum. I gave her a different view to consider, including that some people choose to think, select, and focus on all the negative pieces of information for their own personal reasons, and those things aren't always accurate. I explained that she didn't have to think this way or accept it, because if she surrounded herself with lots of negative things, she'd believe it and eventually become it – pretty much why she was feeling and behaving the way she was. After I had spent some time with this girl, she began adopting a totally different and positive way of thinking – and she certainly kept away from the internet!

Question Twenty-Five

This highlights any other potential and specific issues you might have with diabetes that you can work on changing for good.

Question Twenty-Six

This is about what is important for you. How would you like diabetes to be treated and seen? What can you do to help change this? Does this highlight any other areas that you might need to work on in order to feel better in any way? This can also help with thinking about your personal outcome.

Question Twenty-Seven

Answering this question is really important as it allows you to highlight any limitations you need to let go of in order to feel free and empowered to get what you want from life. The section on Releasing Limiting Decisions in Chapter Five can really help here.

Answering this question can also help you to realize where you should be placing your focus by highlighting everything you *do* want.

Question Twenty-Eight

This question really helps you think about what you *do* want and your own personal outcomes. What personal goals do you have? What would you like to achieve? This is specifically covered in Chapter Nine so you can go out there and get it!

When you come back to these questions again, you'll be able to compare just how far you've progressed in reaching this goal.

After completing this question set, thoroughly work through your answers in the way I've discussed above, and highlight any negative emotions, limitations, traumas, issues, personal goals, and outcomes. Now, as you continue reading through this book, you'll find out exactly how to let go of these issues and the techniques that will help you in doing so. Keep your first answers somewhere safe, so when you go back through these questions, you can measure and compare your success! You've now created a great platform to work from to get some exceptional results.

CHAPTER TWO SUMMARY

- This question set is a great starting point to help you make certain discoveries that otherwise might not be obvious.
- It will provide a good personal indicator of your current health, thoughts, and emotions. You can use this as a platform to work from and clearly measure your progress after applying the relevant resources in this book.
- Answering these questions will help you to spot patterns and make certain realizations that can lead to amazing changes, results, and future comparisons.
- The more honest your answers, the better. You're doing this for you, not for anyone else to judge. The point is to change and improve things for you.
- Reviewing your answers a few times can help to raise additional points.
- Thoroughly work through your answers, highlight everything relevant, and as you read through this book, apply the appropriate resources to address and resolve these.

What Is Diabetes,
and What Do We Mean
By Stopping It?

In a nutshell, 'stopping diabetes' simply means getting our bodies to function optimally and as close as possible to someone without diabetes. As you read in Chapter One, by understanding the mind-body connection, it is possible to take 'stopping diabetes' as far as we wish. That can mean anything from dramatically improving it physically, complete emotional freedom, avoiding and halting complications, right through to reversing diabetes altogether. Ultimately, this is our choice as individuals. Success lies in how we think about our goals, our deep belief system, ambitions, and intended outcome.

We already know the body constantly renews itself and that our thoughts and emotions play an enormous part in our overall health, so there's a lot we can do to stop diabetes and break free right now!

What Is Diabetes Metaphysically?

When we talk about the metaphysical point of view in diabetes, we mean the way our thought patterns and emotional state has created the physical causes that have eventually manifested in the body as diabetes.

No one can answer this question any better than the person living with diabetes; however, from past research and metaphysical study, it is believed that, generally speaking, the probable root of diabetes represents the following: Deep-seated feelings of there being no sweetness left in life prior to or around the time of diagnosis, generally resulting from some form of loss (again particularly at or previous to the time of diagnosis). This often includes longing for what might have been, involving deep sorrow and a great need for control, particularly of something we are unable to exert control over.

This may also involve inflicting some kind of self-pain or self-punishment on ourselves (potentially originating from the general feeling of guilt, particularly survivor's guilt, or a feeling of personal undeserving guilt). It is important to note that the issue of guilt can be unconscious (out of our awareness) until this is really considered or drawn to our attention.

Although this is a general overview of diabetes, there also appears to be the following distinction:

Type 1 Diabetes – A severe loss or shock of some sort that inflicts a lot of negative emotion that is internalized (prior to or around the time of diagnosis), thereby creating a weakened and susceptible immune system. This results in the physical destruction of beta cells and the manifestation of Type 1 diabetes (metaphorically representing the severity of negative emotion and 'loss of sweetness in life'). This tends to happen in childhood and adolescence, because at such ages we aren't able to, or don't wish to, express negative emotions of a particular magnitude.

Genetics and Diabetes Metaphysical Root

For those who have been diagnosed with diabetes from birth, finding a metaphysical cause is actually no different. Life does not just begin outside the womb; the thoughts, emotions, values, and beliefs of the mother naturally affect the development of the foetus. An unborn baby may detect and manifest *all* that the mother is exposed to, thereby determining the physiological development of the foetus.

Looking beyond genetic roots and development in the womb, and going back into the unconscious and engaging our deepest philosophical and spiritual beliefs, there is something more: we must even consider the possibility of metaphysical root causes being carried through a deep core belief in our eternal soul.

This highlights the need to explore your deepest core beliefs when doing this work. Was there perhaps something during your cycle of prenatal development, or even earlier, deep within your soul, that led you to the deep belief or even to experience the loss of sweetness in ways discussed above? Or any of the linked negative emotions?

It can also be the case that a parent has a deep core belief that because they have diabetes, or that it runs in the family, their child will automatically have it, too. This is never a given with diabetes, as only a very small percentage of DNA is actually genetic. If you have been exposed to this type of maternal belief while gestating in the womb, you may have developed this as your deep down belief, too; you may have taken on your mother's belief in not being able to enjoy the sweetness of life for whatever personal reason. In which case, what *do you* deep down believe diabetes is representative of *for you*? Could you have been feeling a lack of sweetness for your mum, or any other reason in the womb?

It's important to acknowledge at this stage that your mind and body are your own and you have the power and resources to change anything you want to. If you find any of this particularly challenging to think about, the section on releasing negative emotions in Chapter Five can help you discover how to work with this and release the necessary emotions.

If you happen to find all this too uncomfortable to consider, you can still use all the other resources in this book to dramatically improve diabetes, so that it never has to be a problem.

Type 2 Diabetes – A loss or sorrow of some magnitude, often leading to stress and depression that can result in an external expression of emotion and looking to external sources to replace the 'lost sweetness' in life (often in regard to particular eating or lifestyle habits) – all of which subsequently leads to Type 2 diabetes. In one respect, a depressed mind or mood leads to a depressed body. It is here where certain conditions begin to develop, as the body begins to adjust accordingly.

It's also worth mentioning that metaphysically speaking chronic illness in general is found to represent fear of the future, not feeling safe, and in some cases a refusal to change.

I would never tell anyone what their particular emotional cause is – and unfortunately, we cannot interview every single person in the world with diabetes; however, based on my own research and that of other professionals, such as Louise Hay, Dr. Tad James, and many others in the field, a consistent pattern seems to be appearing as to root causes.

My own research reveals that the onset of diabetes is closely linked with shock and bereavement of some type. This may not necessarily be death but a separation or loss of some sort that has resulted in much distress, bringing about great sadness or sorrow, combined with guilt in its numerous forms. These emotions may have been unconscious at the time but were manifested internally, resulting in diabetes.

It could be argued that everyone experiences losing the sweetness in life at times, but we don't all get diabetes. However I am referring to this being of a certain magnitude and longevity involving sadness, sorrow, and guilt. For example, someone may appear to have lost the sweetness in life for numerous reasons, but they may not see it this way, or express the particular mix of emotions that appear to manifest physically as diabetes. They may instead feel incensed, life is unfair, and so on, which would physically manifest differently.

Speaking from personal experience, this emotional metaphorical cause certainly resonates heavily with me; it actually confirms what I believed myself when I was first diagnosed. The loss of someone very close and influential to me as a child was a major shock. It resulted in deep sorrow, and I (unconsciously at the time) felt that I could not experience the sweetness of life without having some form of 'bitter pill' to compensate – a feeling of guilt, if you like, that I had my life but this person lost theirs so early. In addition, I was aware of how it affected the lives of close family and felt a sense of guilt, in that I had my life ahead of me but I saw theirs dramatically change.

I think when I look at this carefully, it was all quite thought-provoking and a lot of negative emotion for a child to cope with. As a result, I believe that I ultimately manifested this emotion physically in the form of diabetes, unconsciously creating a sting in my life to feel less guilt about the loss. It is no coincidence that this condition quite aptly represented my emotions and did so for a long time thereafter. You just become more distracted over time, whilst your cells are remembering to hold onto diabetes as a representation of this loss of sweetness.

Using the answers on your personal question set, you can no doubt work out your own metaphorical cause, if you are really honest with yourself and keep 'peeling the onion' until you reveal the core.

Whatever the root cause, the negative emotion – in particular, sadness and guilt –creates a weakened immune system and lowered healing energy, which leads to the physical description of diabetes below.

What Is Diabetes (Physically)?

TYPE 1 DIABETES: Diabetes mellitus (Type 1) is considered an autoimmune condition, whereby the immune system has attacked the insulin-producing beta (β) cells in the islets of Langerhans in the pancreas, so the ability to naturally produce insulin is greatly reduced or non-existent. A person with Type 1 diabetes must inject 'exogenous' synthetic insulin (not produced naturally by the body) or acquire it in some other way (via a pump or islet cell transplant) in order to survive.

TYPE 2 DIABETES: Type 2 diabetes is the result of both impaired insulin secretion and resistance to its action (Type 2 refers to relative deficiency of insulin production). T2 can generally be controlled with medication or diet. It seldom occurs in childhood, but this is known to be changing and becoming increasingly prevalent. Typically, it occurs in adults over 40 years of age.

Although both types of diabetes do differ, the symptoms and the complications experienced have many similarities, as well as the emotional root causes (albeit often varying degrees of these). As a result, it is possible to work in a very similar way to dramatically improve or release both conditions effectively. However, the results with Type 2 diabetes are often much more rapid due to its different physical nature and (usually) lesser severity. I have personally assisted clients in achieving very rapid results treating Type 2 and pre-diabetes, to the point of complete reversal. I have also experienced and seen some phenomenal results treating Type 1 diabetes, too, pointing to potential reversal as well.

Both Type 1 and Type 2 diabetes manifest in similar ways in the body. Without insulin, medication, or any form of control, blood glucose levels continue to rise and lead to the typical symptoms of diabetes. These include excess urination, severe thirst, drowsiness/weakness, weight loss, abdominal cramps, leg cramps, loss of appetite, infection, blurred vision, distortion, confusion, oral or genital thrush, and ketoacidosis (vomiting, hyperventilation, acidotic respiration, and dehydration).

If raised blood glucose is left unchecked over time, or even periods of time, this can potentially damage the small and large blood vessels, leading to serious harm and complications affecting all aspects of human physiology (all the bits that get the well-known widespread negative doom and gloom attention!)

Another effect of high glucose and lack of insulin/medication in the body is the production of harmful acids. A build-up and continuum of such acids results in ketoacidosis, a condition that if not treated with urgency can lead to coma and/or death.

Those with Type 1 diabetes, who must take insulin exogenously, also run the risk of 'over-injecting' insulin, or simply not having enough required glucose in the body due to exercise or not eating enough. In this instance, a condition called '*hypoglycaemia*' (low blood sugar) is induced. As the brain uses glucose as fuel, this condition results in the body being unable to function as usual and results in a hybrid of symptoms, all of which are dependent upon the severity and degree of 'low' glucose levels. The effects on a patient are as listed below (generally, when sugars begin to dip below 4mmol/l or 72 mg/dl).

Effects of Low Glucose Levels	
Autonomic	Sweating, shaking tremors, hunger, pounding heart Palpitations
Neuroglycopenic	Confusion, anxiety, drowsiness, speech difficulty, lack of coordination Atypical behaviour, visual impairment Paraesthesia (variety of uncomfortable bodily sensations)
Malaise	Nausea and headache

People with Type 2 diabetes are likely to have experienced very high glucose levels early on. As this improves, it is quite possible to experience some hypoglycaemic symptoms as sugar levels begin to fall, in order for them to stabilize to a safe level. This is referred to by some as a 'fake hypo', meaning that sugar levels are unlikely to (really) be extremely low (as in Type 1 diabetes). However, it is important to still be aware of these symptoms in case a 'true hypo' was to occur for some reason. 'Fake' or not, hypoglycaemic symptoms are real for anyone experiencing them. Any anxiety can generally be eased by checking the actual sugar level and acting appropriately. In the event of a 'fake hypo', getting a drink of water or having a cup of tea and taking some time to calmly relax with a positive distraction is likely to help. See Chapter Five for appropriate coping methods.

NOTE: Although the following information reported is naturally very dismal, diabetes complications can be avoided, managed and stopped.

In terms of a medically orientated (physical) overview of the complications of diabetes, long-term hyperglycaemia (high sugar levels) affects the microvasculature of the eyes, kidneys, and nerves as well as the larger arteries, leading to arteriosclerosis (hardening of the arteries, the leading cause of heart attacks, strokes, and vascular disease).

According to the *Handbook of Diabetes, 4th Edition* (Bilous and Donnelly, 2010), diabetes is the most common cause of blindness in those of working age, the most common cause of end-stage renal failure worldwide, and the consequences of neuropathy make it the most common cause of non-traumatic lower limb amputation.

However, we can choose to firmly reject the above doom and gloom and take action against this. We need a positive approach, one in which we look to what is good, hopeful, and about all that we *can do*. In other words, do one of two things:

- Wholeheartedly reject the above negative version of events, and focus on all that we *can do* to live a perfectly happy, healthy life, focusing on the real root cause of diabetes and what can be done to resolve this.
- Or, put up with the condition for what it is, fear all of the above, or feel sorry for ourselves, and hope it doesn't really happen to us (something I call the ostrich option – referring to the ostrich's supposed habit of burrowing their head in the sand).

So What *Do* We Want?

As we said at the beginning of this chapter, stopping diabetes and breaking free involves achieving the same blood sugar range as an individual without diabetes, with the least amount of insulin to safely make this possible, right through to fully reversing diabetes and its complications.

Our real intention is to ultimately restore the natural optimum process of glucose metabolism; this will be the focus of visualization techniques covered later in Chapter Five.

Below is a simplified diagram of how glucose metabolism works naturally. Our aim is to re-stimulate this natural process by mentally instructing our existing cells and core physical coding to regenerate new, healthy pancreatic (β) cells.

We already know that other cells within the body such as skin cells can be ultimately reprogrammed to rapidly generate new, healthy (β) cells that are efficiently responsive to glucose (currently evident in mice). We further know that adult stem cells (undifferentiated cells) can renew themselves and differentiate to yield some or all of the tissue or organ of origin – hence an organ like the liver can regenerate itself naturally. This simply highlights what our entire nervous system is naturally capable of; whether we know the full potential of this consciously yet, or not.

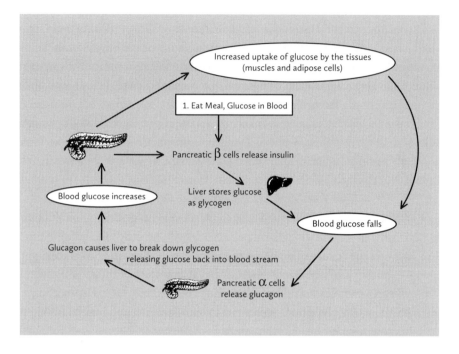

The natural regulation of blood sugar in an individual without diabetes is approximately 4–7 mmol/l, or 72-126 Md/dl, with slight variations on either end of the scale. This glucose level can also be measured by a three-monthly average blood glucose count. This is basically, as it sounds: an average sugar level over a three-month period (approximately). The blood test is based on glycated haemoglobin, meaning a glucose molecule is attached to the haemoglobin molecule (HbA1c). HbA1c comprises the major glycated component in the red blood cells and has been shown in numerous studies to correlate to average blood glucose levels. As the average life span of a red blood cell is approximately 90 days (three months), the percentage glycated haemoglobin is a reflection of glycaemic control over an 8–12-week period prior to the test.

Although there are some factors that can cause minor fluctuations. This test generally provides a good overall picture of control.

The following is a conversion table of HbA1c percentages to average blood glucose levels (the reading we see every day). This will help you with the later interpretation and comparison of results as you see the dramatic improvement and phenomenal changes that will take place as you put into practice the many suggestions in this book.

HbA1c and Blood Glucose Reading Conversion Table
(approximate closest conversions)

HbA1c %(DCCT)	Av. blood glucose (mmol/l)	mg/dl	IFCC (New HbA1c measure)
4	4	72	20
5	5.4	98	31
6	6.9	124	42
7	8.5	154	53
8	10.1	182	64
9	11.7	210	75
10	13.3	240	86
11	14.9	268	97
12	16.5	320	108
13	18.1	352	119
14	19.6	382	130
15	20.6	402	140
16	21.6	422	150

In a person without diabetes, this result would be expected to be between 4 percent and 6 percent. Note, however, that there are different published targets in the UK and USA for targeted glycaemic control for people with diabetes. The National Institute for Clinical Excellence (NICE) in the UK currently suggests a target of 6.5 percent (48) HbA1c and below. Diabetes UK also recommends this target.

The American Diabetes Association, on the other hand, recommends a target of below 7 percent HbA1c. These are reasonable ranges for a person with diabetes to achieve, and such targets are deemed as maintaining very good control; however, these ranges still exceed the normal range expected for an individual without diabetes.

So What Is Our Real Outcome?

My point is that, in order to make any dramatic improvement in diabetes, we need to achieve the same blood sugar levels as a person without this condition, using the least possible additional interventions. Basically, we want to achieve:

- Normo-glucose levels of between 4 percent and 6 percent HbA1c
- A life free from severe hypos
- A life free from being obsessed with diabetes care or living like a saint
- A life free from fanatical exercising or restricted diets for the rest of eternity
- A life free from being a social recluse or party spoilsport
- A life free from injecting lots of excess insulin or taking increased medication
- A normal, ideal weight without compromising or substituting insulin

We want to live life to the maximum and be happy, fulfilled, and healthy, without diabetes being the focal point or a negative distraction. We also never want the potential complications of diabetes to be an issue; however, if for any reason the issue of complications has already arisen, we can manage and work on dramatically improving them too, so they never have to become a limitation either! (See Chapter Eight.) Although the *Handbook of Diabetes* states: 'The overall life expectancy of patients with diabetes is reduced by 25 percent', *I can never emphasize enough: This statement must be strongly rejected, both consciously and unconsciously, as no text has a right to suggest this as a fact.,*

As diabetes is reported to be a rising chronic condition in the world, conventional medicine primarily focuses on its negative implications and suggest and expect the occurrence of such. This sets us up for a medical-fulfilling prophecy, one to be fully rejected. The very essence of this attitude calls for a positive and forward-looking approach in the treatment of diabetes by focusing on the right mind-set to achieve full health and make diabetes (as it is seen and experienced today), a problem of the past.

CHAPTER THREE SUMMARY

- Diabetes has a *meta*physical meaning as well as a physical meaning. This is key in creating positive change.
- Stopping diabetes refers to getting our bodies to function as optimally as possible and as close as possible to someone without diabetes; we can take this as far as we choose from dramatically improving diabetes to reversing it completely.

- Chapter Three provides a specific list of intended outcomes and a blood sugar conversion table to keep track of results and monitor progress.
- Although the potential negative effects of diabetes are often focused on, it is important to concentrate on all that we can do to achieve full health instead.
- There really are no limits as to what we can achieve with the right informed, positive, and pro-active mind-set.

4

The Components of an
Indestructible Mind-Set

Mind-set is everything. It determines our character, the paths we choose, and the results we get in life. Adopting the components below, resources throughout this book, and your own great individualism, you'll always ensure an indestructible mind-set fit for maximum success.

Know That You Are Always in Control of Your Own Mind

If you know that you are in control of your own mind, you'll also know that you are equally in control of the results you get. Although people may often try to control how we think, ultimately we are always in control of this by what we choose to accept and choose to think. An important question here is, if you're not in control of your own mind, who is? If we take personal responsibility for everything we do, we will always be empowered to change things to how we want them. But if we look for reasons as to why we haven't got the results we want, we immediately lose any power to take control and positively change things.

REMEMBER: *Reasons* equals being a *victim*, whereas *self-responsibility* equals *results*. Be confident with this, and take charge of your own mind and results. Reading this book is great proof that you can take control to make positive changes in your life!

Maintaining a 'State of Excellence', Even Through Challenging Times

When I say maintaining a 'state of excellence', I'm talking about controlling what's going on inside in order to control the way we externally look, behave, and respond, thus the results we ultimately get.

This also includes the message we give off to others around us. If we stay conscious about positively maintaining our inner thought process to maintain an inner resourceful state, despite being tired, stressed, or whatever else we are dealing with, we will always be able to manage things better and get the best results possible. The most successful people in the world – be they presidents, emergency service personnel, or Olympic medallists – maintain a 'state of excellence', psychologically and therefore physically, which allows them to achieve distinction in what they do. (I explain this in detail in Chapter Nine, where I describe the steps needed to getting exactly what you want with examples demonstrating where maintaining a 'state of excellence' made the difference.)

Never Be Afraid of Change

We can all change as much as we want to change – when we do, we'll also notice the world around us simultaneously changing, too. Without change, we can't expect to get different results. Positive change is fundamental to life and moving forward. Scientist Albert Einstein summed this up perfectly: "The definition of insanity is doing the same thing over and over again and expecting different results."

Positively Programme Your Mind from the Outset

Before starting our day, it's important to take a few minutes after we wake up to really think about what we want from the day ahead (our outcome for the day). This might be anything from blood sugar levels to achieving something in particular. What do we want to happen? What do we want to achieve? What has to happen for us to achieve this? What can we do to take steps towards achieving our ultimate goal?

When thinking about these questions, get into a relaxed and focused state (more on this in Chapter Five's list of Stressbusters – Peripheral Vision). Accompany this by taking in some deep breaths through the nose and out through the mouth, energizing your mind and body for the day ahead. Strongly visualize these things and even say them aloud: *What is going to happen today? What do I have to do to put this into action?* Then believe it and take action. For more details on working effectively with Goals and Outcomes see Chapter Nine.

Become a Master Reframer – Seeing Negative Stuff Differently

Look to how you can turn negative situations on their head. This isn't to say that bad or negative stuff doesn't happen, but when it does, look at what you can do about it in terms of viewing things differently, and look for alternative meanings. We can do this by:

- Looking for the positive in a situation
- Looking at how you can be pro-active and any alternatives or consolations

- Looking at someone's intention for whatever they've done rather than concentrating on their behaviour
- Finding humour in the situation
- Taking a philosophical view. What can you constructively learn from the situation?

Reframing situations is something I have had to master from a young age, and I can attest that it certainly helps keep you in a strong state of mind, even when negative things happen.

For example, a few years back, I remember having such a severe hypo early one Sunday morning that I went into violent fits, and it took several strong people to steady me. I was in bed, in my birthday suit, soaked in sweat, and shaking uncontrollably. The fits were so strong, I had to be given a rectal diazepam (minor tranquilizer) and came round to find three paramedics and my partner standing over me in my bedroom. Hmmm. If there was ever a time I could have felt embarrassed, that was it! Having had these violent convulsions for some time I was pretty exhausted, too (I've had far lesser workouts in the gym!).

But rather than looking at this episode as embarrassing, and that I should sit around recovering all day, I quickly reframed the situation by joking about the great show I'd just given the paramedics. We got everyone some tea afterwards and had some normal conversation for a bit so that the paramedics were reassured I was fine. It was a good chance for everyone to recover after such an intense situation. I was so grateful, because the bravery, skill, and efforts of one paramedic, in particular, meant I avoided hospital, which would have been far worse. The reality of what they had just done for me outweighed any potential embarrassment.

By the time they left I was naturally a bit tired, but I took my time getting ready and went straight out for a good, hearty breakfast – a great excuse. This was an exceptionally touch-and-go situation. I won't even go into the specifics of what I experienced whilst fitting, but let's say I could have really dwelled on this. Instead, I focused on the fact that I was alive and well and that I could learn from what had happened. Needless to say, I knew exactly what this had been about and, thankfully, it has never happened again. I took the positive learnings from what was a potentially negative situation!

I had to reframe situations when I was first diagnosed, too. I was still a kid, and kids get invited to children's parties, with lots of cakes and buns and other food temptations. I knew I couldn't overdo sweet things as many kids can, but I was still determined to enjoy them. So I insisted on extra time on the Bouncy Castle in order to help get my sugars down enough so that I could have another bun (or two!).

This actually turned out well, because the other kids thought it was pretty cool that I got extra time in the Bouncy Castle, and that whilst they had eaten all the food on offer at once, I still had plenty saved for later. It helped that I had no problem in explaining things to others. I've always found that once people (kids or adults) understand the reason behind something, they can accept it and often do their best to help matters.

When I was slightly older, about age 17 (our teens being a challenging time for many of us), I did have to reframe a little more philosophically, but it still made all the difference. One boyfriend actually said to me, 'You're lucky to have me, because no one else would put up with your diabetes.' This said more about him than me, but I learnt a big lesson about his bad attitude, and it gave me a very lucky escape from a bit of a plank!

Naturally, I was hurt by that kind of thinking, but in reframing the situation I realized that if any future boyfriends were deterred by diabetes, they were never going to have enough metal for my line of thinking, anyway. I certainly wasn't prepared to be manipulated into a relationship by being made to think that I was lucky for someone to put up with a 'diabetic'!

No matter how sinister or seemingly trivial something potentially negative may be, there is always another more productive and beneficial way to look at things. The more we can do this, the better our mind-set and equally, the better our physical health.

Surround Yourself With Positive Influences

It's well known that the people and environment we are around have a massive impact on how we think, feel, and behave. If we hang around someone or something long enough, we often become like them. It's therefore massively important to make sure we're surrounded by positive, supportive, encouraging, and successful people and environments with a healthy mind-set and atmosphere, because this breeds and rubs off. Negativity spreads like wildfire. This is something we often see in the workplace and leads to a very poor working environment, where people survive rather than thrive!

The most positive, successful, and healthy types of people tend to mix with the same sort of groups. Bear this in mind in order to support yourself in the best way possible.

Lose Your Inhibitions – They Serve No Positive Purpose

Inhibitions pertain to a deep-rooted fear of something and only hold us back. Fear serves no purpose, unless it is a natural fear, such as the 'fight or flight' response in the body triggered to ensure our immediate survival; anything else only limits us. Use the resources throughout this book (particularly those in Chapters Two and Five) to become aware of any inhibitions and limitations you may have, and let them go.

Be Willing to Openly Communicate and clearly

The happier and more willing you are to be open about your diabetes, and what specifically helps you best, the better. This helps to cover all eventualities, and to avoid any unnecessary occurrences. Educate the people around you, so they know exactly how to help you, if needed, and in your preferred way. It can also help to have your own preferred resources to hand.

I sometimes worked in a different city at a medical practice owned by a very nice general practitioner. He was aware of my condition, so I was always confident that I was working in a good place if anything were to ever happen (not that I ever expected it to – but I'm always extra vigilant when working alone with clients and not in my own practice).

We were talking one day, and the GP happened to tell me that he had put a tube of Hypo Stop in one of the drawers in the office, in case I ever went low. Although this was a thoughtful (and ordinarily useful) gesture, I personally hate 'Hypo Stop'. It gives me a gluey feeling in my mouth, and I have become incredibly sick from taking it in the past – not to mention that, if I'm going low and anyone attempts to stick their fingers in my mouth, I'm likely to bite them (at the risk of sounding like a certain World Cup footballer!).

I, therefore, realized that I needed to tell him the best way to help me through various stages of a hypo, if anything were to happen and I could not help myself (no matter how unlikely).

I told him about the orange glucagon kit in my handbag (sometimes I just use a quarter measure of the full glucagon to give me that quick boost). I made it clear to only use the glucagon if I'd already gone past the point that he could get me a lukewarm sweet tea and a nice biscuit to solve the problem!

If I'm low, I'm a bit of a stickler for privacy and wanting as much normality or positively distracting conversation as possible. This again was something I had to learn that I needed to tell people.

On a school trip to France when I was about 15, I was dancing at a disco in a big *chateau* where we were staying. Because I was laughing and having a good time, one of my (well-intentioned) friends came up to me in the middle of the dance floor and threw a big bag of jelly babies at me saying, 'Eat those. You're low.' Needless to say, I wasn't impressed, as I wasn't actually low that time. Once again, it taught me that I needed to teach my friend that if she suspected I was low, never to approach me in that way. Instead, she should just simply say that she needed to ask me something, then take me to one side, because if I had really been low, I'd have been pretty upset and annoyed by that, which never helps in a hypo.

By communicating clearly with the people around you, you can create a positive reassurance and outcome for all concerned.

Embrace Mistakes

If we never make a mistake, it tends to mean we've never tried anything new. In fact, we need to make mistakes in order to learn something of far greater value. Constructively learning from mistakes allows us to successfully move on and avoid making the same mistake more than once.

Wholeheartedly Believe In Everything You Do

If we wholeheartedly believe in what we want and do, and have the courage of our convictions, we'll always achieve our goals, because we'll have the motivation, drive, and persistence necessary. There are always bumps and challenges in life, but we'll have the tenacity and patience needed to see things through and find solutions that will get us where we want to go. In this respect, patience and persistence really do pay off, and a strong belief in ourselves will ensure it.

Be You! Free Yourself from Becoming Your Condition

Avoid the 'diabetic' label, and refuse to let diabetes hijack or define you. It gives the wrong focus, and alienates you; you're not a Dalek or any other strange breed! You're a person, so much more than a current condition.

Think Outside the Norm to Adapt and Overcome

Be resourceful and flexible, so that you can find other ways to achieve the same outcome and get exactly what you want. Keep exploring every avenue you can think of. There is always more than one way to do something. Nothing ever needs to stop you, especially diabetes.

Value Yourself and Your Experiences

Whether this includes diabetes or not, knowledge is different from information, as it is born out of experience and character. So it's important to value ourselves and all of our experiences, because these shape who we are, what we know, and who we become.

Our experiences are how we learn, and our character influences what we do with this. It's important to keep learning, because this means we keep evolving and, above all, living. If we don't keep learning and experiencing new things with an open mind, we don't develop and grow; instead, we'll get left behind and wilt away.

Be Confident and Aware, Never Complacent

It's important to be confident and keep a positive focus, but at the same time be aware of everything around us, in order to protect us from becoming 'complacent'. Complacency only leads to mistakes and serves no positive purpose. Confident 'mindfulness' is the key – thinking and planning with a positive focus to ensure we achieve our desired results.

Be a Problem Solver and Utilize Your Unique Resources

Seeing yourself as a problem solver and valuing that ability in yourself is a great way to think about and utilize diabetes. In my experience, managing diabetes can require unique, creative, independent, and resourceful ways of thinking – skills that can be pretty rare in society, as a whole. Valuing these abilities in yourself, and making the most of them, can help you create some positives from your health condition and provide you with some great skills going forward. This includes the ability to multi-task, be more perceptive, remain two steps ahead, be responsible... The list goes on!

I liken managing diabetes to managing a company. If you can manage diabetes well, running a company is a piece of cake (with a cherry on the top, as you get paid for running a company, too!). It's therefore important to value these resources and use them to your advantage. Living well with diabetes can be the driving force that keeps you ahead of the game.

Keep the Imaginary Bee Suit at Hand!

This is a big one. I have seen so many people with diabetes affected by negative comments and insinuations made by medical professionals, well-intentioned friends and family, and those in the media. But when it comes to negativity and limitations cast onto us by others in life, yet another quote from Einstein nails it for me: 'Great spirits have always encountered violent opposition from mediocre minds.'

So avoid, ignore, and reject the 'negi-tudes' (as I call them) like the plague! It can help to pretend to have an imaginary bee suit (the big white protective clothing beekeepers use to prevent being stung). I imagine putting this on if I'm surrounded by negative people or comments; this way the comments can bounce off me, and I'm protected from feeling the sting. This is so important because too many bee stings can kill if we're not careful!

I was going to say that negi-tudes serve no purpose, but on second thoughts I guess they can add to the 'bumps in the road', that we develop new resources to overcome. To really master this particular attribute, see Chapter Five, in the section Dealing with Judgement, and all of Chapter Seven. You'll never look back.

Be Pro-Active, Avoid Dwelling

Avoid focusing on what's wrong, or what you or anyone else thinks something *should* be; instead, concentrate on what you can do and what you do actually want to happen.

Never Let Diabetes, Anyone, or Anything Limit You

Anything is possible, diabetes or not. The only person ever stopping us is ourselves, by allowing ourselves to fall victim to self-limiting beliefs. If you feel you have any of these (and we all do at times), Chapter Five will help with this.

It's often the case that the more challenges we have to get through, the more successful we become, so keep going and be bloody-minded! I've never met or known of an extremely successful person who hasn't had their personal challenges. It's a cliché, but it's so true: that which doesn't kill you makes you stronger. Perhaps this is something to think about when contemplating the purpose of your diagnosis.

Have a Mindful Philosophy – Everything Happens for a Reason

Whatever happens in life – amazing, good, bad, tragic, or indifferent – there's always something we can positively learn from it, and it always happens for a greater purpose in our lives. If we learn to look at what we can positively take from life's challenges in a health capacity or otherwise, this can enable us to get the lessons we need in order to develop our resources and successfully move on.

Champion Your Condition!

Avoid any resentment or pent-up anger over having diabetes, because it can be one of the easiest emotions to experience, especially when things don't always go according to plan. Make the decision to take control, and never let diabetes control you.

Instead of surrendering to diabetes or feeling any negativity toward it, ensure you find what diabetes was *positively* intended to give you.

Develop Awareness of Your Emotions and Their Physical Consequences

It can be easy to dismiss that emotions have a constant effect on our health, but they do, and dramatically, too! All negative emotions correspond to either anger (irritation, impatience, criticism, jealousy, bitterness, resentment, and frustration) or fear (anxiety, nervousness, tension, worry, doubt, and insecurity) – emotions that poison the body.

Learning to be aware of negative emotions, letting them go, finding resolution, and taking positive learnings from them will allow the organs in the body to function properly and avoid creating the negative effects manifesting as ill health. like in the stress cycle. This will significantly improve overall health both short and long term.

Improve Diabetes for the Right Reasons

As a result of all we have had drilled into us about the negative complications of diabetes, it's natural to react by desperately wanting to dramatically improve things. But whilst this is an important reason, it causes our focus to be on the complications and all that we *don't* want.

Choose instead to dramatically improve your management of diabetes in order to be free and live a fulfilled, happy, healthy life. Doing this will create a positive focus and is much more in line with what you really want.

Never Say Never

Always have an inquisitive mind until you find the answers you want. Be willing to ask yourself whether you've got anything to lose by keeping an open mind, applying fresh ideas, and freeing yourself from criticism and doubt. Closing your mind to infinite possibilities only creates limitations and negative emotions that lead to ill health.

The minute we take something negative at face value, the minute we surrender our independent thought and a host of potential opportunities, we are at the mercy of negative emotions. Imagine how depressed I would be if I had accepted what I was once told in the eye clinic!

Explore the Unconventional or Different

Have the courage to explore, understand, and use unconventional ideas in order to make new and exciting discoveries. Often, it is unconventional ideas that provide us with the best solutions, so investigate these.

The more we explore, discover, and learn, the more neural networks we build in our brain, constantly increasing our capacity to think and develop. This enables us to grow as people. Moreover, if we keep growing and personally evolving in this way, we progress to a new level of consciousness, and to quote Einstein one last time: 'No problem can be solved from the same level of consciousness that created it.' Hence we need to have an open mind in order to learn new things and think differently – especially about diabetes and how far we can travel to stop this.

Have a Great Sense of Humour – Laugh When You Can!

If you adopt everything discussed throughout this chapter, in combination with your own great character and existing skill set, you'll develop that indestructible mind-set, which will quickly be reflected in your health, and you'll see your diabetes dramatically improve.

CHAPTER FOUR SUMMARY

- Mind-set is everything. It determines who we are, the paths we choose, and the results we get in life.
- Every successful individual will display these mind-set traits.
- What one person can achieve, so can you! With the right mind-set.

Resources and Techniques

This chapter contains a lot of information and resources. It is useful to read it all, but it is also intended for you to refer to as a personal resource for any relevant solutions you may be seeking.

An Interesting Way to Look at and Think About Diabetes

Diabetes itself is never *really* the problem; it is actually life's various events and how we respond to things that can cause a problem. It is therefore our *response* that results in diabetes playing up, or leads to the manifestation of diabetes to begin with.

It is only when we begin to look beyond the surface of dealing with diabetes and all its implications that we begin to see things very differently. Doing this involves changing the meaning of diabetes to us as individuals, and creating a far greater focus in life that puts 'daily diabetes' into perspective.

REMEMBER: we got this condition for a reason, a higher purpose – to gain the resources we need and move on. Diabetes is metaphorical as much as it is physical. So although the development of this condition signifies a loss of sweetness in life, perhaps going full circle, it was always intended for us to release it (once ready) in order to restore that lost sweetness.

Thinking more philosophically about diabetes assists in pushing and expanding our boundaries to explore new, unlimited possibilities. Ask yourself: Why are you reading this book? This particular section, even? What does it mean in a broader context for you? Are you looking to explore a new way of thinking? Are you ready to move to the next level? Do you need some greater focus in life? For the most profound results we often have to explore and trust in the things we can't always physically *yet* see. If we had never thought space travel possible, we wouldn't have half the knowledge and opportunities we have today.

It all starts with the quality of our thoughts – everything that goes on in our heads. That is what leads to major change! Self-fulfilling prophecies can be positive as well as negative, so changing the way we think and deep down believe is never to be underestimated.

REMEMBER: diabetes is just a descriptive word. You can choose what this means to you. Only you really know what has to happen to change this.

Some Questions to Consider

Thinking differently equals different results, use these questions to reinforce your answers from Chapter Two. These questions aren't meant to be easy for anyone to answer!

- For what purpose did you get diabetes?
- What do you need to resolve in order to achieve total health and happiness?
- What is different now from when you didn't have diabetes (including major things)? Can you spot any patterns?
- Are you ready to let go?
- What does life look, sound, feel, smell, and taste like without diabetes? How does everything seem? Do you like this? Can you make it your focus?

Effectively Dealing With Judgement

Generally, when any of us feel judged (diabetes or not), it is because we feel self-conscious about something, or possibly, that we have a tendency to be quite judgemental ourselves and assume others are doing the same. When this isn't the case and it's a classic indisputable case of judgement, it is always more about the person doing the actual judging than it is about you!

When it comes to judging diabetes (and there's a lot of public ignorance about the condition), judgement can reach a whole new level. One common example I've personally and professionally encountered is people making stupid comments after witnessing someone injecting in public. I always want to laugh and roll my eyes when someone tells me they've had it said to them, because I've had pretty similar myself. It's just crazy, but here goes my little story, and I'm not on my own with this one, either.

I was once injecting in public in a restaurant (a decent one too!), as many people do, and heard one woman say to another: 'Drugs. I can't believe she's shooting up in here, I bet it's heroin.'

I looked at them bemused and said: 'Yeah, because junkies tend to inject into their thigh and test their blood sugar level first … of course, I must be off my head. In future, if you take an educated guess at *insulin*, instead, you might not sound quite as stupid!'

Aside from just being a dim-witted comment, it was more about the woman who said it than it was ever about me. For whatever personal reason of her own, she only had 'heroin' in her head. Perhaps because if she were injecting herself, it would have been heroin – or perhaps injecting heroin is all she's ever seen. Either way, what this *did* say about her was that she needed educating, and some manners to go with it – perhaps even some duct tape for her mouth!

Although this particular incident didn't bother me personally, on a serious note, I know many other people who are far more self-conscious, new to diabetes, and less confident than me who have been affected by such comments. And rightly so, because such comments can still be shocking and insulting. It has put some people off injecting publicly, too, as well as created feelings such as shame and embarrassment around injecting. They end up with a negative trigger and association.

As a result of having diabetes, I've been judged on numerous occasions – worst of all by medics, and inevitably, by family and friends: 'Why didn't you do this?' 'Why didn't you do that?' 'How did that happen?' 'Did you eat something before?' 'Aren't you looking after yourself properly?' And so on. You know the questions that can come, and these only add to the 24/7 responsibility we already carry around, so it's never particularly helpful.

This can make anyone shut themselves off and avoid telling people certain challenges or concerns they may have for fear of judgement or criticism. So all this is to say: judgement really serves no positive purpose. It's important to understand the psychology behind judgement, as well as the importance of self-confidence and having the personal resources to deal with it.

The following techniques and other resources throughout this book will help greatly with this.

Separate a Person's Intention from Their Behaviour

The person's intention is likely to be that they care or worry about you, or they may have some other positive motive, such as wanting to protect themselves (effectively cover their own back, so they don't get into any trouble). To you, however, their behaviour seems to reflect judgement, criticism, nagging, or whatever, and is undesirable.

Generally, people have a personal positive intention for what they do, so focus on this. You might point out to them that you're aware of their positive intention, but their behaviour really isn't helping matters. Help them to realize their behaviour isn't matching their intention, so that they can begin to change it. Further along, I've included some practical examples of this to clarify how this can be used in real life with good effect.

People Only Really See Themselves and Go On Their Own Experiences, Learnings, and Values – Their Own Projections

People reflect outwardly what is inside their heads, based on what they think of themselves or have learnt from experience or their learning. Unfortunately, people often generalize this information and, rightly or wrongly, may apply it to others.

Basically, people are often talking about themselves, their sentiments, or how they might feel or respond in a given situation when they are talking about something. Either way, whatever any of us say or feel, it comes back to some form of reflection on us and all that we perceive. Think about when you were young and playing in the playground. One child calls the other 'Stupid', or some childish name, and the other child says in response, 'I know you are. You said you are. What are you going to be next?'

This is what we call 'projection' – people 'project' what is in their head onto others. Just as an actual projector projects onto the big screen the information that has been fed in, the information that is in a person's head (their thoughts about themselves, beliefs, experiences, and values) is projected onto the recipients around them when a person talks or behaves in a certain way; essentially, the 'recipients' are the big screen.

You can ask the people who you feel are judging you the following questions to help them realize their 'projection' or 'intention', so they can think about it and you can help them to change their behaviour:

- Are you saying this because that's what you would do in my shoes?
- Is that how *you* would feel and act?
- Do you mean that's what *you* really think?
- Have you ever had diabetes yourself, to really appreciate this situation fully?
- For what purpose do you specialize in diabetes?
- What is your highest intention for doing so? (Presumably this will be to make a difference and *help* people. In that case, you can then point out that their behaviour of leading you to feel judged really isn't *helping* you at the moment! This way it should help the person to change their behaviour to meet their intention.)

At a time when I really needed these type of responses to others' judgements, I was too ill to even think of them.

As a student age 19, for example, I was labelled a 'brittle diabetic'. This was attributed to drinking too much alcohol and not looking after myself (which was untrue) and because I was judged by staff to be 'that age'.

If I had been able, I would have asked all the questions above, particularly, 'For what purpose do you specialize in diabetes?' I imagine that I would have eventually got the antiquated consultant in question to say, 'I am a diabetologist to help people.' In which case, I could have responded by saying, 'Well, you're not really helping me by profusely ignoring what I'm telling you, are you?' That way I might have then at least got myself referred to a more useful physician a bit quicker!

Projection

On one occasion, I experienced a classic case of projection, when I was rushed into hospital with pancreatitis and my sugar levels were dangerously high. I was drifting in and out of consciousness when one particular consultant nearly injected me with glucagon (used to increase glucose) until a particular nurse shouted to direct him otherwise. Naturally, with the state I was in, this could have proved fatal. However, when I was eventually stabilized and moved to the admissions ward, the consultant in question went up to my mum and said: 'You nearly killed your daughter today.'

Of course, my mum was completely confused by this, as well as shocked and distraught. It seems some people love to get you when you're already vulnerable. It was only when the nurse came to explain what had just really happened that we realized he was attempting to accuse my mum of something he had just done himself.

The projection was that it was him who *actually nearly killed me* by administering the wrong treatment plan! It was about him!

So, always question what could really be going on in the other person's psychology when you feel they might be saying something negative or unsavoury. Listen to their judgements and comments very carefully to hear what it is they might really be saying about themselves or what's going on in their own head!

Also keep an awareness of times you may be projecting your own negativity onto others. Now that you are aware of projection and have the personal resources to resolve negative emotions, it will hold you in good stead, and you'll be in a much more empowered psychological position.

My examples aside, highlighting the difference between a person's behaviour or projection and their intention leads most people to change their behaviour quite quickly – or at least put a lid on their judgement.

Boot-on-the-Other-Foot Scenario

One of the most useful ways to help a person change their thinking is to use something we call *perceptual positions* – effectively, 'stepping into someone else's shoes'.

Begin by asking the person to just take a minute to consider how they would think, feel, see, and hear things if they were to find themselves in your exact situation by asking them to really pretend to be you for a moment in a specific situation. Really paint the picture for them. Assist them in this by really being as clear and as detailed as possible, so that they can imagine being you.

It is human nature to be pretty self-absorbed most of the time, but if we take the time to do this exercise, we can really begin to see things from another person's point of view. This can give us different and far more productive results from every angle. As we begin to notice things that we might not ordinarily notice, just by imagining another point of view, we can better help the situation. This is effective to do yourself, too. Imagine you were treating someone with diabetes or your loved one had the condition, for example.

Unless they have a personal condition or are pretty all-round exceptional at what they do, most medics and health care professionals don't understand experientially what it is like to live with specific conditions. They read textbooks, attend practicals, see patients, and go to lectures rather than trying to actually feel what it's like to be a patient for any length of time. The 'perceptual positions' technique can really assist with this. It can be particularly effective if you reinforce it by getting health care professionals to apply the technique when thinking about one of their children or loved ones.

Perceptual Positions

When I was in hospital, I once had a visitor who forgot to throw away their empty bottle of juice, and I could not reach it to throw it away myself. A nurse saw it and abruptly said to me, 'No wonder you're in here, drinking stuff like that.'

I was startled and offended by the comment. But as she turned sharply and walked off, I quickly put it down to what she'd either seen before, read, or would have done herself if she had had to manage diabetes – a form of projection of what was in her head but not real. Even so, there's no excuse for such a generalized bad attitude.

Alternatively, if she hadn't had walked off, using the 'perceptual positions' technique, I could have said the following: 'Can you imagine lying here right now (graphically describing how you feel)? Remember: you're here because you've been continually ignored by a doctor, and you are suffering the consequences of that. Then you have a visitor to cheer you up, but he leaves his empty bottle of drink on the side, and you're unable to pick it up. Then comes along a rude nurse who abruptly says to you, "No wonder you're in here, drinking stuff like that." How would you feel right now?'

Then just wait for an answer, followed by an apology, or if not put in a formal complaint recommending a communication course.

The Imaginary Bee Suit Protection

Finally, a great backup in any case of any judgement issues, or off-the-cuff comments that lack critical thinking, is the old imaginary bee suit I mentioned in Chapter Four. Imagine you have one of those big, protective, white beekeeping suits you can put on at any time you need to. Get it out, zip it on, and let any negative or judgemental comments bounce off you as you use any of the above methods to resolve things head on with the person in question.

As I've said before, too many bee stings can kill a person, so it's important to protect ourselves. Never be afraid to use any of these techniques. Focus on the reason you have to use them in the first place. You have the power to change it! At some point, I've used all of these techniques when it comes to feeling judged, patronized, or misunderstood, and they all work very effectively in creating the positive change I've needed. So I hope you find them just as effective.

Beating Burnout

Diabetes burnout is typically defined as the following: 'A state of disillusion, frustration, and even submission to the condition, whereby a patient consequently ignores diabetes for a period of time. Burnout occurs when patients grow tired of managing their condition or prove unwilling to proactively change.'

To paraphrase, it means being fed up with diabetes to the point of being past caring, hence ignoring it for a bit to give yourself a break, which, for a condition that requires 24/7 responsibility, is pretty natural. In fact, psychologically, it would be pretty unusual if we didn't experience, threaten, or seriously contemplate this at points.

Here's the burnout paradox, though: The more someone ignores diabetes, the more it plays up, causes havoc, and requires more attention than before.

Like a dramatic, attention-seeking child (or cat, in my case!), if you ignore them or overlook their initial need, they'll punish you by going the extra mile to *really* get your attention so that you have to notice them. That then takes even more attention, leaving you a lot worse off. Diabetes is no different; it just has far more nasty tricks.

This makes ignoring diabetes as a way of having a break from it far more trouble than it's worth – well, unless you're a glutton for punishment ... and that in itself is something to be mindful of. Remember the question: 'For what ultimate, deep-rooted purpose would you want to cause yourself harm?' That's the only real outcome of ignoring diabetes. In which case, we arrive full circle back at the mind-body root of diabetes being about 'not feeling you can enjoy the sweetness of life'. You would effectively be trying to have a break from your diabetes but actually triggering worse problems. However burnout is about emotion *not* rationale. So how can you beat burnout?

Be Aware and Acknowledge the Signs

Acknowledge the signs, so that you can recognize burnout in yourself and act on it – bring it into your conscious awareness. Also be aware of 'mini burnouts', because there will inevitably be stages on this journey when you might experience little bumps in the road.

There are plenty of resources and advice throughout this book to successfully deal with this. Talk to someone you trust and work out the best plan for you to overcome burnout – because you can!

Be Aware of Your Personal Needs

Sometimes you need a break, but unfortunately just ignoring diabetes is never going to give you that. So what else can you do to give yourself that boost to get back on track and really make positive changes that will ultimately give you a proper break from diabetes? Give yourself another way to let off steam.

Even if it's just for a day, do something to feel free in other ways. Have some fun. Have treats (just inject/medicate accordingly, without getting too hung up on it). Take the day off. Go out somewhere. Do something different – something that helps you to feel free but in a safe and positive way. Even though you still need to check sugars, remain diligent, and medicate accordingly, taking your foot off the peddle a little can make all the difference and recharge your batteries. Visit the coast or theme parks; explore nature; go on activity, leisure, and special experience days; pamper yourself; take a mini break, and so on. Just have some spontaneous fun to blow out, do something different and break routine.

Even giving yourself a day or two in order to do something like this every month, can just shake things up a bit. Create this special time to indulge yourself because you still need to let off steam – just do it productively so it never harms you like burnout!

Create a Far Bigger Focus than Diabetes

I've said it before and I'll say it again: life is for living. If diabetes is your sole focus, you need a bigger purpose to blow it out of the water. There's no reason it should consume your life, and the minute you find something more important, you'll just get on with it. This may be in the context of your career, family, romance, well-being, hobbies, spirituality, education, or business.

What's Your Real Intention with Diabetes?

Presumably, if you're reading this book it's to do something positive and active about diabetes, which you can. This will allow you to emotionally and physically break free, so make sure this is your focus. Allowing diabetes burnout to take over is a seriously flawed strategy; it will only ever set you back. Burnout meets no ultimate positive intention.

What's the Trigger, the Real Root of Burnout?

What is triggering your burnout? Boredom, complications, regimes, responsibility, hypos, self-destruction, external life issues, discontentment, bullying? Nothing is ever as it seems on the surface, and no one just gets burnout without a deeper trigger. You can uncover this by asking yourself the question: 'For what purpose am I so fed up that I don't care?' Then keep asking this question as many times as necessary to get to the real trigger and emotion, which you can then resolve using all the other appropriate resources.

Take the Pressure Off Perfection

Let your ability to successfully acknowledge and deal with your imperfections actually be your perfection, then you really can't go wrong. Remember to give yourself a break and the recognition you deserve in dealing with diabetes 24/7. Too much pressure and expectation upon yourself can have a very detrimental effect and push people in the opposite direction eventually. Accept that there are sometimes bumps in the road, but if you take the positive learnings from them, see them out, and focus on the best you can do about them at the time, you'll be just fine.

Apply these strategies. There's no need for burnout, as it serves zero positive purpose. Choose to take control of diabetes. Avoid it controlling you. You're better than that, and you now have all the resources to go beyond just controlling 'it'. Properly break free and let that be your focus.

Emotional Release Work

In this section, I am going to talk you through the emotional release work as if I am in the room with you, so you can best experience the work. I will give you an online resource to download, so you can listen to this as many times as you need to.

These techniques are based on great successes and continued enhancements gained from working with my clients, as well as combining some of the best techniques that are *also* used within my field. These include, clinical and medical hypnosis (Dr. Milton Erikson), Neuro linguistic Programming (NLP) (Dr. Richard Bandler and Prof. John Grinder), and Time Line Therapy™ (Dr. Tad James), along with the general principles of metaphysics and psychodynamics.

Before starting, it's essential to read through the following important points to get an idea of what I'm talking about and what to expect.

Essential Reading Before Emotional Release Work

1. Never underestimate emotional release work. By this I mean, always be aware of the fact that you'll be letting go of some pretty powerful stuff that has been allowed to manifest and build up over time, so you'll likely be releasing a lot of toxins.

    Depending on your personality and the magnitude of your negative emotion or trauma and how long it's built up, this can mean (though not necessarily) that you may feel temporarily shaky, run down, experience headache, or not quite feel yourself, so to avoid this, please drink plenty of water, keep boosted with good food and vitamins, avoid any additional stresses, and rest well (see the importance of good sleep in Chapter Six).

All negative emotions have to express themselves in one way or another, so be aware of this and know it will soon pass as it leaves you for good.

You'll most likely be fine, just perhaps feel a little tired and/or in a relaxed trance-like state for a little while whilst your conscious mind makes sense of everything you've just done. In this case:

- Get a drink and something to eat.
- Do not drive or operate machinery or do anything that requires focus.
- Rest and allow yourself the time to readjust.
- Distract yourself with something totally different.
- Avoid getting consumed in details over all you've just done, as the mind can also present metaphorical learnings and memories that may not have necessarily happened in reality or be accurately true. However, our minds are very clever and present everything for a reason, so it is important to take all the positive learnings and release the negative emotion using what your mind presents to you.
- Trust your unconscious mind has done the work and things don't have to make complete sense consciously. Everything will integrate over time in order to give you the positive results you seek; usually this happens as you rest overnight.

2. Whenever listening to any of this emotional release work, please ensure:
   - You are in a safe, relaxed environment;
   - You are in the right frame of mind to focus and relax;
   - You are not driving or operating machinery.

3. In the event of feeling temporarily unwell, make sure you carefully monitor blood sugars and inject accordingly. For example, if temporarily you experience raised sugar levels, that is perfectly normal, so administer insulin accordingly or make the relevant adjustments. Alternatively, after some releases, sugar levels can rapidly drop, which must also be kept in mind, so regular eating and monitoring is always important.

Most of my own emotional release work has actually resulted in pretty instant stabilization of between 4 and 5 mmol/l (90–108mg/dl) blood glucose level. However, I have experienced both ends of the spectrum, too, on separate occasions, depending on the specific emotions released. Nevertheless, following these two episodes, the following day my sugars had stabilized perfectly, requiring a very minimal amount of insulin. The important thing to remember is that we're all different and various techniques can take effect intermittently at different times. In a nutshell, just be aware that you will be releasing a lot of emotion, so look after yourself when taking part in any of the following.

4. If you notice any black or dark patches when doing this work, it can sometimes represent quite severe trauma, and this is likely to need to be talked through first. In that case, please consult a professional in the field of psychotherapy to help you address this (see the resource section at the end for relevant professionals.)

5. Where an emotion is extremely intense for you and you feel you are getting caught up in it, allow yourself to rise higher – as if distancing yourself from the scene you are experiencing and ensure you are just watching it from high up above, rather than being in it. Never see the scene as if you are there in it or through your own eyes, in this instance. This is because you would only relive the experience and negative emotion, which is not the intention here. By 'rise higher', you will understand what I mean when we go through the process.

From Chapter One, we know that all negative emotion dramatically affects our health, but it especially has an additional negative effect on diabetes. So aside from adopting a very healthy and positive mind-set, as well as various lifestyle changes, it's pivotal that to dramatically improve and stop diabetes, we first work on releasing any negative emotion, stored trauma, or limitations.

IMPORTANT NOTE: Although I will be taking you through all the emotional release techniques at the online link, I am unable to respond specifically to your needs personally. Therefore, if you do find you need further assistance, please seek a suitable practitioner, such as a good hypnotherapist, psychotherapist, or NLP master practitioner or trainer by asking if they specialize in 'releasing negative emotions'.

Releasing Negative Emotions and Limitations

Once you get used to these techniques, they are likely to become easier. You can use them as many times as you like and also as a very useful resource to have for the rest of your life. Eventually, you'll be able to take the basic principles of these techniques and apply them at the drop of a hat. This way, you'll get the same results in terms of effectively releasing negative emotion any time necessary in the future.

In completing your question set in Chapter Two, you'll have particularly highlighted certain negative emotions, traumas, and limitations that are most relevant to you, and it is important to work on these specifically. We must also remember that there are often emotions underneath emotions. For example, for a long time, I thought that I was feeling extreme *sadness* about something; however, underneath this, I was also experiencing *fear* and *guilt*, as I mentioned at the beginning of Chapter Three. It's therefore important to consider all key negative attachments and work on releasing *every* associated negative emotion.

In this respect, there are only ever two real emotions in the world: *love* and *fear* – the latter obviously being the negative emotion. This is because whatever negative emotion you may be experiencing, if you really analyse it, it will come down to a fear of some sort.

As discussed earlier, a 'natural fear' refers to something we all need: a flight-or-fight response in order to protect us from harm. All other fear is useless and harmful to us in terms of our optimal health and well-being. As well as the emotions particularly significant to you, it is vital to let go of 'unnecessary fear' – the fears that serve you no positive purpose. For example, even *anxiety* and *nervousness* ultimately pertain to fear.

Before you refer to the actual technique, please read the reminders about the process below on what to expect, and how to ensure a full, positive release. However you experience this is great – some people may sense, feel, or hear things rather than necessarily 'see' them in this process. So take what your mind presents to you. Trust yourself.

Important Reminders About the Process

- When instructed to 'take the positive learnings', always ensure that these are *only positive*. Even if this takes some consideration, take the time to make sure you get them all and find the positives – what are the learnings you needed to take at that time in life from that event? Pause the audio at that point if you need to.

- Acknowledge that some experiences that your mind may present to you are metaphorical and may not have occurred in reality. However, it is important to work with what your mind presents for a reason. So go with this, but avoid dwelling on it. Take the positive learnings from it, and release any negative emotion that it signifies.
- Be confident that you are not deleting any memories, but you are simply removing the harmful, unwanted negative emotion attached to it.
- Ensure you are only observing the event from a distance in order to fully take the positive learnings so that you can release the negative emotion? You must ensure you are a good distance from the actual event, so that you have a more objective eye. Make sure you are only observing the event and are *NEVER* in it, so that you can distance yourself from the negative emotion.
- Ensure you are definitely at the very first event in which you first ever experienced this negative emotion. If you are not, then drift further back to this time, and trust the part of your mind that knows when this was. It doesn't have to make sense to you consciously!
- If you experience extreme upset and feel too emotional when looking down on a particular event, ensure you rise your balloon higher and keep rising upwards in order to distance yourself from the emotion. Keep going with this, as you need to release the negative emotion.
- Ensure you have definitely taken *all* the positive learnings you can. Are there any more positive learnings you can take in order to release *all* the unnecessary negative emotion? What do you need to learn before this can happen? Really push yourself here! Remember: positive lessons only, so you can use them for your future success, coping strategies, and safety.
- Have you fully blown away *all* the old negative emotion? Make sure you obliterate every single molecule of negative emotion. If you have *all* the positive learnings, you will be able to do this, because it has no purpose!
- Ensure you fully understand how there is no point in the negative emotion, that it serves no purpose and it's only bad for your health.

It only prevents you from healing, full health, and happiness, and you want these things, don't you?

- It's often natural to feel a little dazed following this technique, or you may feel a little tired. Either way, this is perfectly normal, and it is best to either relax, rest, or get a drink and distract yourself with your usual business, trusting your unconscious mind to integrate all the work you've just done.
- All releases are different and personal. There is no right or wrong experience, and you don't have to feel a dramatic difference to experience fundamental change or for the process to have worked; we're all different in this respect.
- Always ensure you have released the right negative emotion. Ask yourself if your particular trauma or event could in fact be linked to a different emotion.
- Always drink plenty of water when engaging in any release work in order to rid your body of any built-up toxins that have manifested, and rest accordingly.

A Final Note Important to All Release Work

Please be aware that the direction of the past for you may be different. Whatever direction you feel your past is in, this is fine, and go in that direction when you are prompted to turn and face the past.

This is also the same when referring to your future. It is always important to follow what your mind presents to you. If you are unable to visualize events well, then you can feel, think, or listen through the process. The point is to do this in the most appropriate way for you, in order for it to have maximum impact. The key in any of this work is to take what root events your mind presents to you and to take *all* the positive lessons from this that you can, in order for you to effectively release any negative emotions you are working on.

Before starting this process you will need to answer the following question very quickly so that it comes from your unconscious mind. It does not matter what the answer is; just take whatever your mind presents to you in an instant. Trust yourself throughout this process. This could even be something in a past life, or in the womb (as mentioned in Chapter Three), as much as in your current lifetime. Avoid focusing on any accuracy; take an instant answer and trust this – sometimes the mind works metaphorically.

- What was the first event in which you ever experienced 'x' negative emotion?
- When was this period of life?
- How old were you?

Please refer to the audio download to experience this complete process, so that it will make sense. Keep listening to the audio and read over the reminders to ensure a good full release!

> **For the actual release of negative emotion technique, please visit www.dr-em.co.uk to download the audio and do this with me as you listen.**

Now you know this process, use it regularly to take out negative emotion when it occurs. Now ensure you repeat this process for every other negative emotion you highlighted from your question set in Chapter Two, as well as removing all 'unnecessary fear'.

For Any Limitations You Have

Anything that prevents you from doing something or having a happy and fulfilled life, if it isn't an apparent negative emotion it is generally a limitation, a limiting belief, or a limiting decision that you've made at some point in your life that is having a current negative impact on you. For any limitations you have recognized, simply ask yourself:

- What is the root cause of me adopting this limitation? What caused me to adopt this limited thinking and belief?
- When was this?
- What was the decision I made at this point that caused me to develop my limitation?
- What negative emotion was behind this limiting decision?

Important Note About Attached Negative Emotion

Remember most limitations also pertain to unnecessary fear if you track this back far enough. Some fear is necessary; it is there to protect you, so you will naturally never get rid of this. For example, a fear of jumping off a cliff is natural, as it will save your life. The removal of negative emotion only pertains to those that are not appropriate to the situation. For example, if your pet got run over tomorrow, it would be natural for you to be sad, even devastated and upset. It is when this becomes a continually extreme or manifested negative emotion that it is a problem and needs to be released. For instance, if this sadness created dis-ease or prevented you from functioning or enjoying life, it would be a problem. Otherwise, certain negative emotions are natural and need expressing in the most appropriate and safest way to let them out, such as having a good cry, punching a pillow, blasting it out in the gym, running, cycling, and so on – whatever is safe and helps you best!

> **For the Release of Limitation technique, please visit www.dr-em.co.uk to download the audio and do this with me as you listen.**

The basic premise here is that everything in life (good or bad) happens for a reason; it is only when we can gauge and comprehend this reason and learn from it that we can understand it differently. In that way, we can release it in order to rekindle opportunities and embrace our life differently. That's because we are able to realize the positive lessons we need from it.

After that, holding onto any life limitations or negative emotions is pointless, as it only creates a needless negative spiral that harms our health or limits our life.

Resolving a Particular Trauma or Phobia

When we experience a particular trauma or any form of distressing situation, it can imprint in our minds and subsequently manifest physically or psychologically as panic attacks, numerous bouts of illness, or post-traumatic stress disorder, potentially destroying our health as well as critically impeding our quality of life.

Although it might seem ironic, I have come across several individuals who have been in quite a dilemma with their diabetes because they have a needle phobia! So you can see how certain phobias can quickly cause a life-threatening challenge. It's also the case that most phobias in some way relate back to an initial trauma at some point in a person's life, hence they manifest it as a phobia.

To prevent this we can apply certain techniques to help desensitize and decode a particular trauma or distress – basically, eliminate the old related feelings to such experiences so that our mind begins to process them differently. This helps by removing the negative charge associated with the negative situation and replacing it with different positive feelings. We begin to see our traumatic experiences differently, as we don't view them in the same light as before. We attach different associations and meanings to them that prevent the physical and psychological distress or current phobia from continuing.

As mentioned before, any way you feel most comfortable doing this process is fine. It's always important to take what your mind presents to you and work with it. There is no right or wrong way, as long as it works for you.

Please also apply the points discussed in Important Reminders in the Emotional Release section, as these also apply.

If you are going to release a phobia, you first need to ask yourself when your phobia first developed and what it is related to. You may know the answer to this instantly, in which case follow the audio, referring to this connection as your trauma.

If you are unsure of what the root cause is, then it is in your unconscious mind or you wouldn't have developed the phobia. In this case, you can ask yourself very quickly *'What is the root cause that triggered this phobia?'*. Take the first answer that comes to mind, but you must do this quickly to avoid thinking of an answer consciously.

If you still struggle with this, you might want to directly consult a hypnotherapist, NLP practitioner, or psychotherapist for help. Either way, take action to remove your phobia, as you never need to suffer from this as a problem. It is important to note that *if you suffer from any form of phobia that makes this release model challenging or uncomfortable, there are different ways to release your phobia,* so you can either contact a relevant practitioner, or release fear as your negative emotion generally, before you begin.

For the Release of Traumas and Phobias technique, please visit www. dr-em.co.uk to download the audio and do this with me as you listen.

Congratulations on any emotional release work you have done! Any releases of negative emotions or limitations will serve you well in relation to your overall health, and it's a huge part of improving and stopping diabetes! All the techniques above will dramatically help with this, when worked through properly.

Releasing Stress and Depression

Stress and depression are obviously harmful to anyone's health, but both can devastatingly impact diabetes, leading to a vicious cycle if we don't put a stop to it.

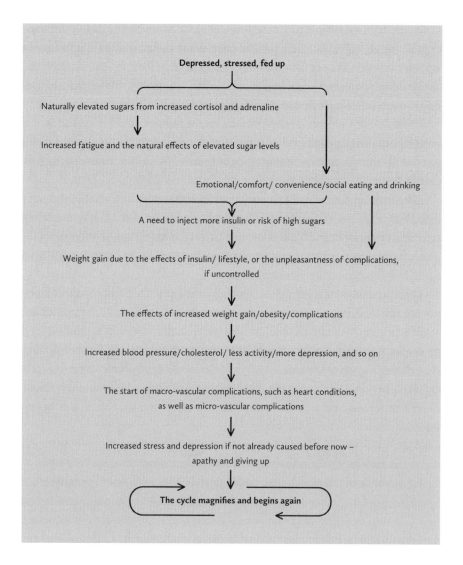

Diabetes is one of those things you can't ignore, even if you try – remember the 'burnout paradox'; it only gets worse. So suggesting you can be in denial of diabetes is ludicrous! However, it is possible to be in denial of the real problem behind it and, unfortunately, diabetes management often gets the brunt of this, hence the incorrect labelling of 'diabetes denial'. Whatever the real issue behind any of the above spiral, whether this relates initially to diabetes or not, it can soon wrongly get labelled as a diabetes problem, and therefore never really gets treated properly.

It's critical to target the root cause of any depression and stress by using all the emotional release methods given above and below. If you're unsure of the root, it can help to start by persistently asking yourself the following questions:

- For what purpose does 'x' make me feel this way? What is the negative emotion connected to this? For what purpose and why?
- What has to happen in life for me to enjoy it and feel fulfilled? How can I get this? What can I do?
- What is my purpose? Who do I want it to be? What sparks something within me?
- When was the last time I felt happy, healthy, and well? What has changed since then?
- What roots do I really need to look at? Are there any deeper issues behind these that need addressing?
- What is blocking me? What do I need to release?
- If depression was personified, who or what would it be?

By working through these questions, you'll eventually arrive at the core root issue you really need to address. You'll then begin to see things from a different level of consciousness – more philosophically. You'll be able to get a better perspective on things, as well as take the right action to solve the problem creating the depression.

We already know that stress directly results in higher blood sugar levels, and depression seriously disrupts good diabetes management. We all experience stress during different periods of our lives. No one is immune, and how we deal with it can make all the difference. Below are some techniques that will help you effectively deal with stress and depression in the best way possible.

The Resources – Releasing Stress and Depression

We can use the neurology in our brains to naturally support our ability to self-calm and successfully tackle stress and depression.

Anchoring

Anchoring can help bring about positivity and calmness by creating a natural, automatic link between a particular physical action or object and a specific positive feeling in the body. Once you've created this link, you can then apply the physical action/stimulus at any time, and it will automatically evoke the positive emotions linked to it. This is an effective, quick, and simple technique. Examples of familiar *anchors* (also called *triggers*) are music, particular scents, or tastes.

Hearing a particular song on the radio might automatically evoke a certain memory, emotion, or period of time, for instance, or tasting a particular food might trigger a specific feeling that you automatically associate with that taste. For example, when I taste strawberry Nesquik milkshake, it takes me back to when I was 10 years old and in hospital, after I was intentionally sent low in order to experience a hypo for the first time.

Scents can also be a strong trigger. If I smell lavender, for example, I automatically think of being about four years old and in my grandma's garden, collecting lavender leaves. Lavender stimulates a very calm and happy childhood emotion in me, so that would be a positive anchor I could utilize.

Alarm clocks are anchors for a lot of us, because when they go off, we automatically respond by knowing it's time to get up or act in some way.

Finally, anchors or automatic triggers are used regularly in advertising to make us naturally connect something to a particular product. Often this can be music. Mobile phone companies, for example, use current popular music to create a constant reminder of them.

An anchor or trigger is a particular physical stimulus (an object, music, taste, smell or action) that automatically stimulates a certain response in how we think and feel; it evokes certain emotions, memories, and associations, causing us to respond accordingly. This then naturally affects our state of mind – either positively or negatively.

We can use positive anchors to help with stress or depression. We can create our own positive anchor and evoke it at any time to induce calm and positive feelings. Anchoring can be used to help change our state of mind – and of course, the results we get.

How to Create a Positive Anchor

1. First, close your eyes and take some long, deep breaths (inhale through your nose and exhale through your mouth) to slow down your breathing. As you relax and your heart rate slows, feel the oxygen flowing easily throughout your entire body as you begin to relax deeper and deeper, allowing all other conscious clutter to float out of your mind.

2. Now remember a time when you were really relaxed, calm, confident, content, and happy – perhaps on a lovely holiday, in a spa, the garden, or whatever works for you. When you think of that time, see it through your own eyes as if it were happening right now.

   - *See* the things you *saw.*
   - *Hear* what you *heard.*
   - Really *feel* the *feelings* of being calm, relaxed, and confident.
   - *Smell* any apparent *scents* of your surroundings – especially if it's the fresh sea air, grass, sunscreen, flowers, food, and so on.
   - *Conjure* any *tastes* you may have had.

Use all your senses in this way to experience that time again, as if it is happening right now.

3. When you are engrossed in this experience and totally reliving it, when it is at the most intense point, snap your thumb and first finger together tightly.

4. As soon as your feelings start to lessen, release your fingers and open your eyes, feeling calm and relaxed.

Now you have just created a positive, calm anchor that you can use whenever you are stressed to automatically induce those positive feelings.

All you have to do is snap the same fingers together, and your neurology (*the nervous system, your mind and body*) will be naturally stimulated to create an association with the positive feelings of the experience you initially linked to this action.

If other triggers work better for you, such as scents or music, you could spray or rub a particular scent onto a piece of cloth/handkerchief you keep with you in a pocket. You can use it to stimulate positive feelings, whenever needed. Sometimes, I wear a particular perfume because it reminds me of a happy memory in a favourite place of mine and I always feel positive, calm, and happy when I wear it. Similarly, you could download a certain track of music to your phone that you can easily access if it has a similar effect.

My partner even has a suit 'anchored' to an extremely successful presentation and feelings of powerful confidence. Use whatever works for you. Have fun with it, and work out what works best for you. We're all individuals, so never be afraid to experiment.

You can use the anchoring technique for other feelings, too, such as being *motivated, excited*, or *energized.* Use a different finger as your association for each one, or some other easily accessible point on your body. Make sure it is in a permanent place, one that does not move about, and that you can easily remember and access the point or object.

If you want to generate several different positive triggers at once, add or 'stack' them on the same anchor point – for example, the finger and thumb action. Just do the above process several times, each time using a different but positive emotion. For example, individually anchor a time where you couldn't stop laughing, then a time when you felt really confident, followed by a time you were really motivated, joyful, happy, content, and so on. Whatever you choose to use and however you choose to do this technique is great. One caution, however: Avoid overusing your anchor, or you may need to keep refreshing it.

Another Resourceful Technique For Dealing With Heightened Stress

- Breathe as suggested above (*in through your nose and out through your mouth*).
- Relax your arms, shoulders, and neck, allowing this feeling and wave of calming relaxation to spread throughout your entire body.
- As you experience or think about the stressful event, imagine stepping out of your body and seeing yourself in the scene (like you're watching it as a movie).
- Begin to see it through someone else's eyes, someone neutral, watching it all unfold on CCTV.
- Then swap and look at the situation from the other person's point of view. *Really* step into their shoes.

NOTE: It's important to get fully into the mind and body of someone else. Use all your senses to do this. Delve into their life and their line of thinking (their likely values and beliefs). Really imagine having their situation.

This simple technique will help lessen the emotional impact by taking the charge off your own personal feelings. It helps you gain perspective and puts things into context, because you are no longer so personally engrossed in the event. It can even make certain situations seem quite amusing (or even trivial), depending on your sense of humour, and of course, the particular situation you're involved in.

A good example of applying this technique is if a family member may be causing you a particular challenge. See them for the *person* they are, rather than the *relationship* you have with them and the expectations that go with this. Take Mum or Dad, for example. All of us naturally have certain expectations and needs we want met by our parents, so those times when their behaviour does not match our personal expectations can heighten our emotions, the situation, or our stress levels. By *disassociating* (disconnecting) from the family relationship for a moment, and seeing our family members as ordinary people, things can start to look and feel very different to us – more normalized and offering a different perspective on the incident. We can question that if they weren't our parents, would what happened seem as unusual or as upsetting? This technique can help, take the 'emotional charge' off the situation.

For example, if my parents do or say something that irritates me a bit, I put it down to them having a 'Mardy Marc time' or a 'Clare moment'. Equally, if it's the in-laws, it might be an 'Irate Irene' or a 'Dicky Dave' attack. Well, you get the picture... It just helps to lighten things up a bit, put them into perspective, and even remind ourselves that we all can have our moments.

If you really get into *being* them for a moment – with their background and values (and if you don't know this, perhaps learning about it will help matters) – you can often begin to see things differently once again. Whatever your relationship may be with the person – whether they are your senior, peer, or junior – their inner child sometimes comes out. Along with other factors, this can help us look at *why* they might be behaving in a certain way, rather than simply looking at *how* they are behaving, and thus prevent us getting aggravated by their behaviour.

All this is not to necessarily condone a person's actions, or say that their behaviour is acceptable; however, if we focus on *their intention* (the real reason behind what they are doing or saying), rather than their undesirable *behaviour*, it can help with understanding the situation and person – and most importantly, lessen our personal stress.

Certainty is a key human psychological need. We may not be able to predict other people's behaviour and actions, which can cause us stress, but we *can* be certain of our own response and how we choose to feel about the situation. With practise, we can be prepared and cause ourselves far less stress – or hopefully, none at all.

Using the above effective techniques to cope with stress and anxiety will have a very positive impact on your health, in general, as well as help you improve diabetes and manage challenging situations in the best way possible. Skilled therapists, particularly NLP practitioners/ trainers and hypnotherapists, can assist you with this, if you feel you need a helping hand. Use what works best for you in order to obtain the best results, and keep practising/ reading over the techniques as many times as you need to.

Understanding Stress – If We Get it, We Can Do Something About It!

Why do we allow ourselves to feel stressed by something? There may be a host of reasons, ranging from personality clashes and individual underlying root causes, right through to having a deep-seated fear of something.

But these are only niggling, superficial reasons for feeling stressed; the deepest reason is far less personal, in fact ... because it's the same for us all! If we keep asking ourselves *'why'* we are stressed and *'for what real purpose'*, we eventually get to the same core reason:

> Ultimately, we all just want to live happy, free, and fulfilled lives, according to our personal values, and something more superficial is preventing us from doing exactly that – something that conflicts with our innermost values (according to our personal model of the world; hence, there are numerous varieties of stress).

This *something* then becomes our *'preventing factor'*, which ultimately pertains to the *'root cause'* of stress, because we see it as preventing us from getting what we really want in life, thereby causing frustration, anxiety, apprehension, anger, and various other negative emotions that result in stress. Such stress results in a series of other negative health consequences, causing the negative spiral to continue, as we've seen in Chapter One. What follows are some important resources to assist in eliminating this.

The Stress-Busting Techniques and Tool Kit

As you already know by now, I've never been a stickler for living by strin-gent rules, because it can really hinder flexibility, and I happen to believe *flexibility* is one of the key ingredients to succeed in life. One philosophy I'd happily live and die by, because it's so true and it's critical in achieving what you want, is the following:

> *'Focus' on what you do want, what you can do, and what really matters for the best results. Have an 'awareness' of all else.*

So, whenever you are feeling stressed, ask yourself: *For what purpose am I stressed?* You'll no doubt get a string of reasons, but for every one of those reasons ask yourself further: *For what purpose?*

Keep going with this question, until you get to the answer of wanting 'to be happy, free, and to live a good, fulfilled life'.

Then stop and think for a minute: *Is the superficial or momentary reason for me being stressed really going to prevent me from ultimately getting hap-piness and fulfilment or achieving my important goals in life, or is it just an inconvenience that needs a bit of creative thinking and flexibility to overcome it?*

Ask yourself how you can be a problem solver with the issue, instead. What would you advise someone else with such a challenge? Do you have a contingency plan, if needed? What else can you do if 'x' should happen?

Whatever the answer may be, it's important to make the decision to take personal responsibility for your own life and look to *what you can do about it and how best you can manage something,* rather than worrying about what you can't do or what won't happen.

Importantly, there's a big difference between 'focus' and 'awareness', and it's crucial to be mindful that we need both. Our focus is where our energy and attention are predominantly directed; however, our awareness is what keeps us mindful of all else going on in our life, enabling us to remain re-sponsible and safe as we 'focus' on the right things. This way we can see beyond the stress and keep our mind on what counts. So, all that we do want will come to us a lot easier and quicker.

In a nutshell, focus on what you *do* want, rather than on what's wrong. Get used to finding the positives of a situation and how you can move for-ward from it. Although challenging to find at times, there will be some positives you can take and things you can constructively learn. Just have a good search, and think outside the box.

Always ask yourself what message life is trying to give you, how can you overcome obstacles, and what it is you are really working towards? What is your real intention, beyond the immediate stress?

Keep your focus on this answer because, as we have discussed in this book, what you wholeheartedly focus on, you will attract more of back to you. So if you home in on the negative things, you'll attract more negativity back to you, and the cycle will only continue – basically, giving rise to the common belief that things happen in threes or 'It's just one thing after the other'. Alternatively, home in on the positive things, and attract more positivity back into your life. Naturally, it's important to appreciate that you can't just think something and have it happen – that's just misunderstanding the principle. To ensure you have the right focus in place, see SMART goals in Chapter Nine.

What you sow (in terms of your deep-seated values and belief system), you reap! This is based on the principle that 'like attracts like' in terms of energy.

From experience, I'm sure you already know that if you deep down expect something, it happens. That's because we programme ourselves to fulfil this by either consciously or unconsciously giving that expectation our devotion. We then get it – good, bad, or indifferent. So truly believe in what you want. Have conviction. Go for it. It does, and will, make an enormous difference to the type of results you get!

If you expect to get stressed about something in particular you likely will, because you're focusing on the wrong things. Work to change this, and focus positively on your intention for doing something in the first place by using the above questions and considering other ways to reach your positive intention where necessary.

Awareness and Reprogramming

It's important to be able to recognize when you might be starting to feel stressed and anxious, so that you can begin to apply the above techniques. Notice what happens in this situation. Is it just a feeling? Do you experience a physical reaction, such as stomach-ache, headache, extreme tiredness, toilet trouble? Does your behaviour change? Do you shout or cry easily?

If you struggle to recognize changes, it may help to keep a regular diary of your feelings, and look for any patterns and triggers that you need to work on in order to eliminate or address the root problem; you may be unaware of this consciously. Similarly, if you are close to someone and trust them, you could ask them to gently point out little changes in your behaviour they notice happening when you begin to get stressed.

Develop an Ongoing Sense of Humour to Keep a Positive Focus

The more we can avoid taking ourselves too seriously the better! The more things we can find to laugh at and become good at 'poking fun' and 'friendly banter', the more this will help us to relax.

This is because humour and laughing actually alter our physical state. The release of endorphins (feel-good brain chemicals) triggers more positive thoughts and feelings. This in turn allows us to focus more easily on what we *can do* to resolve our stresses, rather than focusing on the problem, which only results in bad feelings, hinders our thought process, and contributes to more stress.

Laughing alone helps induce the release of endorphins, which naturally elevate our mood and feeling of well-being. Even making a conscious effort to smile can actually help change your mood. Try feeling down or angry whilst smiling or laughing (see the Rob the Ripper example in Chapter One). It's pretty hard. So always keep in mind the expression on your face and positive body language. (There are more specific information and tips on developing a 'physiology of excellence' in Chapter Nine, in the section entitled The Keys to Success.)

Even 'pretending' to be calm and happy, will help alter your mood and lead to clearer thinking, which will help you solve the problem causing you stress in the first place. Pretending to be, or doing an impression of, someone who is overtly comical or calm can also really help to get you into that state. Even singing aloud in a theatrical musical style about why you're stressed can help to make things seem different, less serious, and change your thinking about it – or at least help you to relax a little by expressing things in a different way. In this way, your state of mind begins to alter, so you become more resourceful and productive.

Lee Mack (a famous British comedian) does a funny sketch where he sings in musical style an argument he had with his wife so the heated disagreement doesn't seem noticeable to the kids while they are on the train. It is hilarious, and also shows how an argument can be made funny, lessening the negative feelings or stress (depending on your type of stress). It does work.

Fully Immerse Your Head in Water for a Few Seconds

Fully immersing your head in either warm or cold water for a few seconds is said to reset the amygdala (the part of the brain that deals with emotion). This can change your focus to a more positive one by refreshing you. With a clearer head, you can begin to see things differently. This will help give you the serenity and fresh, clear thinking to confront the root cause of the stress in a new way, so you can do something proactive about it.

Take a Two-Minute Timeout

Another simple technique is to take a two-minute timeout. It may be simple but never underestimate it, especially as it is so effective but we often don't take the time to do it.

Take two minutes to sit down and do some deep breathing (it's an old and perhaps obvious one, but it does really help when done properly). Inhale deeply through your nose to fill your lungs to maximum capacity and then exhale deeply through your mouth. Do this several times, and stop if you become dizzy.

Now, close your eyes and remember your favourite place – a place where you were relaxed, calm, and having a good time, perhaps a lovely holiday/relaxation day/fun scene, or the like, and just indulge for a few minutes. See what you saw, hear what you heard, and really feel those calm, relaxed, fun feelings. Alternatively, if you created a 'positive anchor' earlier, apply that now. Or use the Unwinding Motion technique described below. This will help to bring back some calmness and help you think more clearly by changing your state, which as we know, seriously affects the results we get.

Unwinding Motion Technique

The following visualization activates the mind-body connection by using all your senses to create positive changes.

Stop for a minute. Close your eyes, and ask yourself where in your body you are carrying the stress, nerves, or anxiety you are feeling. Give it a colour, a size, and a shape.

Now, shrink the area down, seeing it get smaller and smaller, so small it's able to travel throughout your body to an exit point, such as your hand (so you can open it up and throw it); your foot to kick it; your mouth or nose to exhale or blow it out; or any other bodily orifice you might choose to use to let it exit your body. As it's travelling to the exit point, see the colour getting increasingly faint, and as it becomes fainter and fainter, feel the stress, nerves, or anxiety becoming less and less intense.

Now take this small, faded shape, and release it from your body, so that you fully *release it* and *let it go.* See it drift into oblivion. *Physically feel the release.*

Now, have a good stretch and shake it out. As the feeling of stress releases, retune your focus, and do everything necessary to tackle the real root cause of this particular stress to ensure it stays away for good!

A Good Question Set To Ask Yourself

The art of self-questioning can really help to get things into perspective when feeling stressed. In some cases, it can even dissolve the problem altogether. Simply by getting to the heart of the matter, looking beyond the immediate problem, and using a process of deduction (gradually breaking things down), we can often see how some things aren't really a problem at all. Ask yourself the following:

- Does it really matter? Is it really that important in the grand scale of life? Is this stress really worth sacrificing my health for?
- Although a little drastic sounding: If you were to die tomorrow, would there have been any point in being so stressed and wasting time over it?
- Would it matter or make any difference if you did or didn't stress about it?
- What is stressing really going to achieve, if something is going to happen anyway? What's the best, most productive action you can take to get the best possible outcome given a situation?
- Is your focus in the right place? What is your main purpose and intention for doing something? Is stressing helping this and creating the right focus?
- How specifically is something a problem? What is preventing you from reaching a solution? What resources do you have available to you?
- Are you being as resourceful as you could be in the present situation? What can you do about it?

Peripheral Vision

Whenever you're stressed, you are, of course, experiencing various forms of negative emotion, whether this be anger, frustration, fear, or guilt. A useful technique to help alleviate this is to send yourself into a relaxed and calm state called *Peripheral Vision*, which helps with focus.

This technique is very simple but amazingly effective, because when you are immersed in the state of peripheral vision, you're unable to access any negative emotion at the same time. This allows you to get on with what you need to do, without any stressful, anxious, or nervous distractions, and calmly perform at your best. It's also important to keep practising this state for the best results; practise makes perfect, and when you are doing it right, it will work.

Here's how you get into the peripheral vision state:

- Focus on a particular spot in front of you, above eye level. This could be a picture hook, a light switch, an alarm, or the like – anything above eye level.
- Now notice everything about this spot – the colour, size, shape, what it might look like if it wasn't there, the purpose and function of the spot, and so on.
- Whilst still focusing on this spot, expand your vision outwards 180° either side of you whilst still looking at the spot. Notice what is beside you, what you can see in your peripheral vision whilst looking at the spot above eye level. Notice all the things you can.
- Repeat this process as many times as necessary to ensure you are in a relaxed and focused state. You can also heighten this experience by inhaling deeply through your nose and exhaling through your mouth.
- Now, bring your eyes back down to eye level, and carry on your regular business in a much calmer and more centred fashion – one that allows you to get on with things and be far less stressed, if at all.

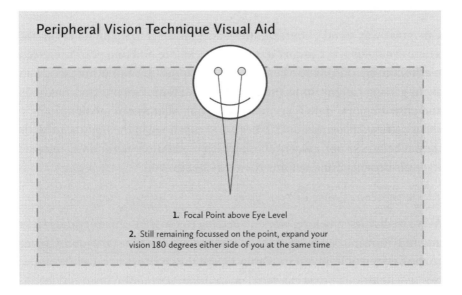

Engage in Regular Activity and Take Yourself Out of the Situation

When you are feeling stressed, activity may be the last thing on your mind. At such times, though, it can help enormously if we push ourselves to engage with normal activities, because it helps release endorphins (the brain's happy chemicals and natural painkillers).

Make sure the activity is something you enjoy, and that will encourage and motivate you, even if it's just a short walk to a coffee shop, sexual activity, or walking to your newsagents or post office, instead of driving, or parking a distance away from the supermarket entrance to walk a bit further, and so on. Never underestimate the power of fresh air and changing your environment and surrounding yourself with positive people to free your mind and generate endorphins.

Even picking up the newspaper, reading a magazine or a good book, or calling a friend can be a great distraction to help readjust your focus and take yourself away from the immediate situation.

Often being in the same environment that the stress or problem is created in, or in which it is experienced, causes an automatic association between the two – like the anchor or trigger we mentioned earlier. Therefore, it will always be more challenging to solve a problem and feel differently if you feel confined to, or stuck in, the same environment as the stress or problem was created. So metaphorically, as much as physically, it's vital to break out and free ourselves, whenever we can!

Explore Meditation

One great way to take yourself out of a situation is to meditate regularly. There are many ways to meditate, so just explore and find your preferred method (more on this further on in the chapter). It's important that you avoid getting caught up in the specifics of different meditation methods and obsessing over details (as many often do). All forms of meditation help reduce stress and benefit overall health, as explained in the Body Scan Meditation below. So don't worry about which meditation method you choose; if it feels beneficial and helpful, then it's right for you.

Tackle the Root Cause of Your Stress

As we've discussed before, work on getting to the root cause of your stress and fully understand what it really is all about. If you're struggling to get to the bottom of it, invest in seeing a good therapist who can assist you in this and help you release the problem or negative emotion once and for all. Although it can feel like a daunting prospect, it's well worth it, if you work with the right practitioner for you.

Take Action and Trust Yourself

Be flexible and resourceful in your actions and trust yourself, because you already have the answers; you just have to get into a resourceful state to find them. Relaxing and changing your scenery will help with this. It's crucial that when you get to the root cause of your stress that you take the necessary, practical and realistic action to deal with the problem in order to eliminate subsequent and superficial stresses once and for all.

Separate Intention from Behaviour – I Will Say It Again, Because It Really Helps

If a particular individual is the so-called instigator of your stress, it's important to separate their intention from their behaviour in order to deal with it. In other words, find out the person's intention for acting or behaving in a certain way, rather than focusing on the negative behaviour they are displaying. If you do this, you are likely to find their reason for acting a certain way, even if you have to ask them specifically what their intention is. You can then act accordingly in the best way to help them to change this behaviour (see the Dealing with Judgement section for more details on how).

Here is an example of separating intention from behaviour. Say your child has been shoplifting. Whilst this is a bad behaviour that you might well be stressed about, look at the intention behind their actions – perhaps they have to shoplift to protect themselves from being bullied by another group of kids (a positive intention for them). Once you've separated intention from behaviour, you can work out precisely what positive action you can take to do something about it. By addressing the root cause, you can eliminate it.

Confront the Problem

Even when other people are involved, it is still our responsibility as the person experiencing stress to look at what it is we can do to control and positively change the situation. The person with the most flexible behaviour in doing this always controls the situation, because they are willing to adapt and use whatever appropriate resources necessary to get the best results.

For example, if your stress is to do with undue pressure from your boss at work, confront him or her and make your feelings clear, but always state your own intentions for doing so.

For example, if the boss is making demands on you in order to get you to do extra work and bring in more money for the company, then subsequently your taking sick days as a result of the stress would defeat that intention, as sick days are expensive and cost money rather than make money.

In such a situation, you might say: 'I'm feeling very stressed about *your current demands*, which leads to me feeling unwell. Unfortunately, this will result in me needing time off work, if it continues. This obviously won't help anyone and runs counter to your initial intention, which was the source of my stress in the first place. I am fully aware of your intention, so if I can just get on with my work as productively as possible, it will serve us all best.'

If you still feel you're not being listened to, look to what else *you* can do. Have you considered changing companies, working for yourself, a change of career, studying something new, getting what you need to enter management yourself? Either way, use all your resources to confront the problem to solve it.

Write It Down or Talk It Through

Writing things down or talking things through with someone helps to externalize things. It can take some weight off your mind, as well as help you see things in a different light. Sometimes, when you see things written down or hear them said back to you, they often don't seem half as bad as when we have them whizzing around inside our heads.

Use a List

Listing things can help us see the problem in other ways, what we need to do to be proactive in solving it, as well as create extra space in our minds. Make two columns on a piece of paper, one column for 'problems' and one for 'solution options'. Write down all of the problems that result in stress for you. Write next to them all the possible ways to resolve and solve them. Although some options to solve the problem may not be desirable or necessarily easy, they are nevertheless an option to resolve the root stress and serve you better in the future for when you're ready to let go and confront them.

See this as a 'solution action list', and work through it a bit at a time to avoid any overwhelm. Do what you can, when you can. Everything is a positive step forward, and you'll ultimately feel better for it. Tick off each problem once you've blitzed it. If you can carry out a little task every day that allows you to make progress in sorting out a problem, things will soon change in a big way, and it will also help you keep your attention in the right place. It's important to reward yourself for taking action – give yourself other incentives to keep going and keep motivated (even if something small).

Problems Causing Stress	Solution Options	Action
Money Problems	Extra work/debt consolidation/ family help/	✔
	Sell Items/ Citizens Advice/ social help, and so on	✔

Generally, there are so many resources to assist in stress relief that are very effective; however you may find some work better than others, depending on the particular cause or type of stress. If you follow the simple pointers above, you'll soon begin to think and feel differently. More importantly, you'll experience a massive difference in sugar level stabilization, because effectively **stress = sugar.**

The Benefits of Meditation

Even if you're good at dealing with stress, it can be beneficial to have other ways to relax, eliminate anxiety, and use your mind. You might already be familiar with the power of meditation, or it might be something you've never considered or even written off as something only Buddhists and hippy types do. But it's something anyone can do, and it's a great skill to learn and keep practising. It certainly sharpens the mind and aids mental focus.

The particular meditation I'm going to explain is one that is particularly useful in improving diabetes. As I've mentioned, there are many different ways to engage in meditation, as it simply involves different ways of using our minds and beginning to experience phenomenal results!

Scientific studies show regular meditation can:

- Lower blood pressure and improve circulation
- Increase energy and creativity
- Strengthen the immune system
- Release stress, fatigue, and toxins
- Lower blood glucose levels
- Extend our life by approximately 10 years
- Aid in looking and feeling more youthful
- Provides more psychological rest than a full night's sleep from just thirty minutes meditation.
- Aids decision making and productivity.

The Body Scan Meditation that follows is a great way to get started using your mind in the intended way. Whether you see yourself as a novice or an expert, it's helpful to keep some tips and reminders at hand to get the best experience you can.

So before we begin, here are some general pointers:

- Find a quiet, isolated spot, free from distractions such as television, telephone, and computer.
- Meditate in a pleasant, clean, and tidy environment that you can relax in.
- Take time to get into a comfortable posture for your body, so that you can fully relax and enjoy the experience.
- Take time to empty your mind before starting. If you find that your mind is just too busy, you may want to do a couple of things first to help clear it. Exercise is helpful, so is asking yourself if you can attend to all else in your life later and allow it to wait. Imagine you are allowing all your stresses and concerns to just float out of your head with every breath you exhale, and temporary shut it out. Then go back to meditating. If you're really struggling avoid forcing it, because the time to meditate isn't always right, and you want to avoid creating a troubled experience.

- Breathe deeply and slowly during meditation – in through your nose, to fill the bottom of your lungs, and out through your mouth, long and slow, until you empty your lungs again. Avoid forcing or rushing the process. Also be mindful to stop if you feel dizzy from this.

- Meditating first thing in the morning or last thing at night are considered the best times, because our consciousness is in an altered state, making us more receptive to utilizing the mind-body connection. Plus, if you're like me, you'll no doubt be here, there, and everywhere, being busy throughout the day. So these are excellent times to meditate, unless of course you're on nights, in which case, listen to your body and choose the times you feel relaxed or naturally trancy to meditate.

- Experiment to find the most comfortable place and method to meditate. Once you've found this, use it as often as possible, as you'll create a positive association that will make it easier and quicker to get into meditation thereafter.

- Meditation is a personal process, and there is no one right way to do anything, other than what's right for you and what gets the results you seek. So have confidence in what you choose to do, and enjoy it.

- Whilst meditating, it can sometimes be helpful to have light music in the background. This music can be whatever relaxes you and creates calmness. Alpha wave music can be particularly helpful in getting you into the right meditative state (see box).

Alpha Wave Music – Certain music that you can purchase specifically helps you get into a relaxed meditative state. It is called *alpha wave music*. This type of music can be helpful because when you successfully meditate, your brain waves naturally alter and you enter a deeper level of consciousness. This is what's known as the *Alpha Level*, which allows for positive meditative results. Often a particular challenge when meditating is to stay in the alpha level long enough to avoid distractions like mental chatter, lack of focus, or physical restlessness, so certain music can really help with this. A particular music I've used in the past is called *Omharmonics,* which I found to be a pleasant version of binaural beats to nicely guide you into alpha level. However, anything that helps you personally in your meditation is just fine. Music isn't essential at all, unless it's your preference.

When to Momentarily Leave Meditation

When you feel down or depressed. This is because intense focus and concentration may increase receptivity to negative thoughts and attention, when something deep hasn't been dealt with or resolved. So first change your focus to something positive, retune your thoughts, and shift into a positive mood and feeling by remembering or imagining a time that you were at your happiest, using your anchor or trigger, as discussed earlier. Work through all the tips and techniques previously given in this chapter, then enjoy meditating. Remember: practise makes anything better.

Leave it if you've had too much caffeine, recreational drugs, food, or alcohol, as this may influence your mental focus and ability to relax. It's also best to leave if your sugar levels feel unstable in any way, to avoid distraction or frustrating confusion in this state.

Body Scan Meditation for Health

This method is simple and can be conducted on its own, with other forms of meditation, or as prescribed mind-body work.

- First of all, lie down and begin calming the mind, using the deep breathing described above.
- Repeat a short mantra (language pattern) or positive affirmation (such as to improve specific health or achieve a specific desired outcome). Focus on what you want to happen. Here are some examples:

Anxiety mantra – I am safe and free to enjoy life. I have a choice. There's always something I can do, and I trust in the process of life.

Diabetes mantra – This moment is filled with joy. I deserve to enjoy it. I can and I will enjoy the sweetness of life. I'm fit, healthy, and well, restoring my cells and natural balance in metabolizing glucose.

Depression mantra – I create my own life. I deserve to enjoy life and do what I can. I deserve to have what I can in life and appreciate this.

- Once the mind is calmed and focused on what you want, focus on your breathing, feeling it rise and fall throughout the body.
- Once you have become in tune with your body, focus on your left toes, feeling the sensations in them over a period of 20 seconds or so.

- Following this, expand attention onto the sole of the foot, and stop to notice the sensations felt there.
- Feel the energy in your feet, and visualize this, giving it a colour and shape, even a temperature.
- From there, direct this energy and attention around the body – up the left side and down the right side, allowing the colour, shape, and temperature to become increasingly prominent, glow, and expand in size.
- Finally, focus on the torso, gradually feeling sensations rise through the neck, face, and crown of the head, paying particular attention to the face and head.
- Feel a sense of well-being around the lips and eyes, specifically the areas that relate to smiling, which, as we know, intrinsically promotes happiness.
- Finish by focusing on your breath, as it falls from the crown to the navel and rises again in several cycles back and forth. During these relaxing breathing cycles, make positive suggestions to your mind and body, to activate the changes you seek and/or apply the mantras above.

NOTE: I will discuss a specific suggestion pattern you can use when we get to the section on Reducing Blood Sugar. For now, just know that you can add to the effectiveness of this part of the meditation by visualizing clearly the desired changes, especially regarding health and healing, that you want for your body. It's important to warm up to the process of doing this meditation and become comfortable with it. The more you practise, the easier it will become, and you will notice more and more profound changes – from increased relaxation to vastly improved health. Enjoy!

Releasing Anxiety

Anxiety is one of the most common feelings. We all experience it from time to time, whether we have diabetes or not. Feeling anxiety often signifies that we fear something. This fear can sometimes be a good thing. It may motivate us to do a good job, for example, and to remain conscientious due to the fear of reprisals – or if we turn this round, wanting to do the best possible job for all-round fulfilment.

But feeling anxiety can also signify that we have an extremely irrational and intense fear of something that begins to limit us and becomes debilitating. It's all in the reason behind our anxiety and how we utilize it.

Anxiety is something I have had to manage as long as I can remember, diabetes or not. It is something I have to regularly question myself about, to distinguish if something is really a problem or not. It keeps me very focused and has made me articulate in carrying out any job or task I do, which I have been able to use to my advantage.

In this respect I now refer to anxiety over wanting to do a good job as *positive* anxiety, as it gets the best out of me. For *positive* anxiety, I then changed the meaning of negative sensations like knots in my stomach to represent charged-up positive energy and excitement that I am ready to release, instead.

However, there have been occasions in the past where I have experienced *negative* anxiety with an intense fear behind it, which has been essential to distinguish, so that I could successfully eliminate it. In fact, most anxiety can be crippling and extremely limiting, so what follows are ways we can resolve this. Some important questions to ask yourself to get to the bottom of your anxiety are:

- What's behind this anxiety?
- What can I do to resolve it?
- What needs to happen in order for me to become anxiety free?
- Is it my mind simply telling me to keep focused on what I'm doing, alerting me to do a good job, and be conscientious because I want the best?
- What would happen if I wasn't anxious? Does this serve any purpose for me?
- What is this anxiety? What does it mean? What is it teaching me?
- If anxiety was a person, who would it be in me?
- What's the alternative feeling to anxiety that I'd prefer?
- What's stopping me from feeling this?
- At what times am I not anxious?
- What are the differentiating factors between when I am anxious and when I'm not anxious?

Whichever way we look at it, anxiety is generally our unconscious mind telling us to focus, and we have to respond accordingly to resolve it. What follows are several different ways to resolve different forms of anxiety. Most other techniques mentioned throughout the book are also useful to apply here, in which case I will direct you to them.

Work Out the Root Cause Behind Any Anxiety

Use the question set above to do this, and tackle it to fully resolve the issue. Make a clear and specific plan of what you can proactively do, and take action toward this.

Acknowledge Anxiety Itself As a Good Thing

Your mind is alert and simply telling you to focus – and that you need to do something and act. Either way it is protecting you. Even people who are excellent at what they do get nervous and anxious before they perform. You just have to ensure you channel this in the best way possible by turning it into positive energy ready to release through the action you take. This comes down to your focus and deep belief system – what messages you give to yourself.

A Technique to Help with Anxiety Messages

In your mind, fly into the future, just after the specific event you are feeling anxious or nervous about. Clearly visualize a big success, something that signifies you've done a good job and achieved the outcome you want.

Make sure you really get into this. See what you can see through your own eyes (as if you are experiencing it right now). Hear the things you can hear. What are people saying, what are you saying to yourself or others? Finally, really feel all the positive emotions you can feel – all those great, warm, and satisfying feelings. Use all your senses, even appropriate tastes and scents that are present. Really go for it – no holding back on your success!

Now lock this in your mind, right there in the future. Seal it in tight, so it stays right there. Stick it down, lock it in, and throw away the key!

Now come back to the present and keep focused on that successful outcome awaiting you.

REMEMBER: What you focus on, you attract, so keep it positive. Keep seeing the outcome you want, and take all the practical, realistic actions necessary to achieve it! It's important to acknowledge that as much as we visualize something, we must still take the necessary practical steps to achieve it.

For example, when I was first ever invited to teach a training course by myself in the Emirates, I visualized clearly a great success; however,

I still had to do all the preparation necessary to make this happen, such as projector slides and excellent course content, and so forth, in order to achieve success. By visualizing success, I knew my intended outcome, and this ensured that any anxiety was expressed as positive energy, allowing me to perform at my best, rather than forgetting my words or messing up the delivery of the excellent training sessions I had planned for my clients.

IN A NUTSHELL: Strongly visualize what success after the event will look and feel like, and perform the necessary steps to ensure success. If you do that, then you will successfully transform any anxiety you are feeling into positive energy to ensure successful results.

Engage the Universal Law of Attraction

The more you focus on success or positivity, the more you will attract it to you. I know you know this by now, so work it to your advantage in every way possible.

Be Prepared

As much as possible, plan ahead to avoid any potential for anxiety, and give yourself peace of mind. If you know you have measures in place, you can relax. Teach yourself that you can let the anxiety disappear right now, because it serves no purpose; it's not actually real or tangible, except in your mind. You can choose to re-create your reality any time you wish.

Reframe

If you feel anxious, take all of the steps above and say to yourself, *Stop!* You might even use a positive resource anchor, as described earlier; for example, anchor a positive time, when you felt the opposite of anxiety, deflecting any negativity and changing it to a positive way of thinking. Ask yourself, *What else can this mean, and how can it help me see things in a different light?*

Reframing to Avoid Anxiety in Certain Situations

A different example of reframing can be used when you are perhaps feeling anxious about having a hypo if you're going out for a walk, driving, or doing something, such as competing in a sport, public speaking, and so on. If this is the case, the following can help:

Keep Ahead of the Game With Provisions

Although it can be perfectly natural for blood sugars to drop during exercise, if this does happen, we want to avoid having to endure any dangerous or unpleasant side effects, because if we're prepared we can control this all the way, and it doesn't have to happen.

Take action and plan ahead to ensure that you have a pleasant walk, or whatever the event is. Pack enough medication, sweet snacks – say, ones you would enjoy anyway, even if you didn't need to eat them (so it's no great shame). Have a bite to eat before you leave, or slightly reduce your insulin beforehand, so that you have something to burn off.

Always pack a glucagon pen for additional peace of mind, and make sure someone you are with would know how to use it (although instructions are included – it just saves vital time). Alternatively, if you're alone and it would make you more comfortable, drop it into conversation with someone where you're planning on going. This is about focusing on a positive solution but having awareness of a potential challenge that has been causing unnecessary anxiety so you can resolve it.

Avoid Overthinking Things

It can be all too easy to overthink things. In some cases, certain things are going to happen, whether we like it or not. Often when we overthink things, it plays out far worse than it actually is.

It can help to air your feelings with someone else (making sure they obviously aren't worriers or pessimists themselves – because negativity breeds). Talk about what you are *really* anxious about, beyond the immediate cause. Focus on some positive self-talk, and take things one step at a time. Simply live in the moment, rather than think about what *might* be or what's possibly ahead. Take it as it comes, and deal with it *if and when* it does happen.

As I've mentioned before, if (God forbid) you died tomorrow or became seriously injured in such a way that it changed your life, would this overthinking really be of any significance? Couldn't it just be a complete waste of good time and energy? Isn't life for living and enjoying it? In which case, if you spend it overthinking and worrying about it, what's the point in being alive in the first place?

Model Your Preferred State

Think of a person you deem responsible but carefree and confident, who just goes for what they want and gets on with things. They may be someone you know, a television personality, film star, comedian, or the like. Now, imitate their traits (never to be rude, but just to take on board their positive attributes). How do they go about things? How do they hold themselves? Copy their posture, attitude, and their line of thinking, as if you were almost doing an impression of them.

See how simply 'modelling' someone else for a bit can actually change and uplift your own behaviour. After all, what you practise, you become. This can also help you begin to distance yourself from your own nerves and anxiety until you can fully release them (as preferable and discussed earlier).

Dealing With Anxiety During a Hypo

I hate the 'anxiety' stage of a hypo, but I also know it's my unconscious mind working to alert me to do something quickly – basically, to consume sugar to balance my B.M. This is actually something to be thankful for, in a very strange way.

Obviously, preventing is far easier than curing a hypo, as we all know, so all the planning and preparation we discussed above is worthwhile if it prevents not only 'hypo' anxiety but anxiety, in general. Diabetes can, unfortunately, still sometimes catch us off guard – I liken it to the naughty child that plays up from time to time – in which case we have to deal with it and assert who's boss!

Here are a few important pointers that have proved extremely helpful in hypo situations:

- **Make sure other people are trained by YOU to best help YOU** –
  Make sure that those who you spend time with and who live with
  you know exactly how best to reassure you in the event of a hypo.
  Ensure they know to stay calm and treat you normally, whilst
  helping you by getting you a sweet drink and snacks, or injecting
  GlucaGen, if necessary. It can help for them to place sweet snacks in

front of you, so that you feel more reassured that sugar is available and you will soon be fine.

As we can display a variety of emotions and behaviour in a hypo, regard for *you* as the person behind this is critical. It's important for others to know that although a person might be 'low' and their 'conscious' senses may be a little distorted, their subconscious is still highly receptive. It *all* goes in at the unconscious level, and that's what leads to additional physical reactions and future feelings we may have (such as future anxiety), without always consciously knowing why.

Beyond the conscious mind, we always remain aware and can easily detect stress and panic in others. This can therefore project onto us, provoking additional responses that could otherwise be avoided. This never helps in a hypo situation, so make sure people know the drill, especially your preferred drill.

- **Find the most suitable place possible** – If you're out and about, find the calmest place possible to sit down and sort out the situation, preferably somewhere with fewer people buzzing about, as additional and various types of noise can really add to anxiety. If you're in familiar surroundings, settle in the calmest place that generally allows you to feel good – it can act as a positive anchor! Sometimes messy, noisy, or particularly warm rooms can add to hypo distress.

- **Avoid constant blood sugar testing when low** – It can be easy to want to keep testing blood sugar to see if it's gone up; however, it can sometimes take a while before the results actually show up on the monitor, although you may feel more stabilized. In this case, just concentrate on fully recovering rather than constantly checking, as a lower number than previously shown can naturally cause increased anxiety (because the sugar hasn't fully filtered to show this on your reading yet – in other words, it's a superficial reading).

  This is also important to acknowledge to prevent eating too much glucose as a knee-jerk response. This way you can avoid going too high later. From experience, I can say that this is a very easy mistake to make, so trust yourself and how you feel as much as a B.M. machine reading. Be sensible about testing, but space it out.

- **Make sure others know to share B.M. results** – If other people insist on checking your sugar levels, because you are unable to, make sure they know to share the results with you and remain transparent.

  For example, on several occasions, I've reached a particular 'low sugar' level but insisted to my partner Johnny that I'm okay and feel fine, despite him telling me otherwise. So it actually proves of enormous benefit to show me the figures in black and white, so that I can't contest it. This simple action has tended to calm me down and help the situation, getting me to act or accept help.

  Seeing your results is an important point, because it can add to anxiety if you feel like you don't know what's happening – especially as hypos can leave you feeling extra anxious or out of control, as it is. So if people know to work *with* you rather than *over* you, this can help make things much easier and help to reassure you.

- **Use distraction to help overcome unwanted anxious feelings** – Once you've acted in terms of getting the sugar you need, or you're even in the process of waiting for your sugar levels to rise again, familiar distractions can really help to take the charge off any un-wanted feelings.

  I like to put on the television or play some music where possible, to normalize things and distract me, or for Johnny to tell me about some work issue or discuss some light family-and-friends news whilst I recover, as this really refocuses the mind. Recovery tends to happen much quicker and faster then.

- **Avoid overwhelm when low** – In any situation, *overwhelm* (think-ing about too many things at once and getting stuck in unnecessary details) really creates extra anxiety, so it's important to focus on one thing at a time – the big picture.

  Focus on dealing with the hypo, and to hell with all else. Things will easily be sorted out later, because everything seems complicated in a hypo, as you'll know.

  Make sure others know to reassure you and remind you of this, as well as that they can help you catch up with things later. Basically, have them reassure you that other things aren't a problem. This way you'll avoid getting negatively distracted or frustrated with them. I'm sharing this point because so many times I have found myself going around in circles, getting frustrated because I've tried to think about all the other things I've got to do. I've even started to try and work out accounting details when I've been going low. In my experience, this has only ever led to a really anxious type of hypo. I've then fully recovered and had no idea what I was fussing about – it was all easily sorted out, when I could think straight.

In mind-body medicine, the metaphysical significance of hypoglycaemia tends to be 'overwhelm' about something, so perhaps this is something worth thinking about and looking for your own hypo patterns.

All of these points can certainly help in dealing with hypo anxiety, but you'll find some of them work better for you than others, because obviously going low and diabetes itself is a very personal experience. Work with what is best for you, as it helps alleviate unnecessary anxious feelings you may have.

Resolving Emotional Eating

Emotional eating is something we've probably all been guilty of at times, from being bored and reaching for something tempting and naughty to eat, or being upset and scurrying for the chocolate, or being fed up and calling to order a takeaway – even being lonely and going to a drive-through.

We all eat emotionally from time to time; it's about recognizing it, and being self-aware enough to distinguish if it's a regular pattern that's harming you and needs to change, or whether it's a one off you're fully aware of and perfectly entitled to! Either way though it is important to have appropriate strategies in place to deal with it effectively, especially if it is a bad habit that can be damaging to your health.

1. Ask yourself, *For what purpose am I going for this?* Really. Be honest!
2. If there is a person behind your emotional eating? Who could it represent?
3. What emotion is behind it? Is my eating this piece of cake going to solve the emotion?
4. What else can I do or have in replacement?
5. What has to happen for me to get satisfaction elsewhere other than from junk food? How else will I be content? What action am I going to take to achieve this and change things?

114

6. Use the following positive mantra: 'I'm more intelligent than this. I know how to solve this challenge without simply trying to eat it away. I care about my health, and I can do better than this.'
7. What positives am I *really* getting from emotional eating? Am I just self-punishing?

Answering this question set will help you recognize emotional eating and change it where necessary, as you now have the resources to deal with any negative emotion behind it.

Tackling and Ditching Dia-Bulimia

Whether we're talking about bulimia, anorexia, or 'dia-bulimia' (the latter just being another label to describe how someone can be experiencing bulimia through using or manipulating diabetes), they're all a condition surrounding body image and weight loss for a particular reason.

These individual labels relate to the process used to manipulate food intake. This may be binge eating and purging afterwards (bulimia), starvation (anorexia), or a bit of both in relation to injecting minimal levels of insulin (dia-bulimia), for the same outcome – weight loss, body image, or feeling more comfortable in our own skin.

All are a form of self-harm, related to deep-seated unhappiness. And when it comes to diabetes, all are extremely harmful to our health – long term as well as short term – which I'm sure you've already figured out.

There's usually a time in life (diabetes or not) when we reach the point of wanting to lose weight. But as anyone with diabetes doubtless already knows, it is never quite as simple as just exercising and restricting calories.

By dramatically reducing insulin units, irrespective of whether you eat or not, you'll lose weight. This is because when insulin isn't reduced naturally in accordance with the right levels needed, the body begins to break down muscle tissue as well as inducing continual vomiting, ketoacidosis, and severe dehydration. So whilst it might be a quick, sure way to lose weight, it's sadly got devastating repercussions that aren't even worth the weight loss.

It is a false economy, because the consequences of such actions will inevitably result in numerous hospital admissions, which will in turn result in weight gain from the excessive amount of insulin that will then be pumped into you – never a morale booster. A vicious cycle then continues until you become aware of this and decide to break it – which you can easily do!

A clear decision needs to be made at this point. Do things differently and more slowly, or open the door to becoming an amputee, blind, beset by constant infections, and so on – you know, all the 'potential complications'. Those potential complications unfortunately fast become 'inevitable complications' if we engage in a continued cycle of 'dia-bulimia'.

The good news is that this can be avoided. There is a lot we can do to resolve the roots of 'dia-bulimia' and deal with any complications that may have crept in, as well as safe and effective weight loss.

While dia-bulima can be seen as a 'quick fix' to weight loss, it's also a 'quick flop' because of the deadly repercussions; otherwise, we'd all be at it! So unless anyone's trying for a super skinny coffin, knock it on the head or avoid it like the plague now you're aware of it. Unfortunately, dia-bulimia is no genius solution to weight loss!

So What's the Solution? What Can We Do About It?

Stopping dia-bulimia really depends on every individual's personal reason for instigating it in the first place, so see what best resonates and act accordingly.

- **Self-harm** – Ask yourself for what purpose you or someone you know is self-harming? What has to happen to make you or them care enough about themselves to stop? Dia-bulimia is a very cruel form of punishment or physical display of unhappiness, a desperate cry for help and attention, so the root cause needs tackling and fully resolving. This way you can get to a good positive solution!

- **To look good and lose weight** – There are just as effective ways to lose weight, such as dramatically reducing insulin in such a way that it does not result in high blood glucose levels that cause the problems of 'dia-bulimia'. On the face of it, reducing insulin but still being able to eat what you like may seem attractive. It would to anyone, let's be honest. So no one can judge that one, if they're being straight with themselves. But the repercussions are far from pleasant, never mind the long-term implications.

  In this case, it becomes about stopping a habit and gradually increasing insulin again carefully and steadily, as any rapid changes can potentially bring about complications. You may also be more sensitive to higher doses of insulin and at risk for severe hypos.

Once glucose levels return to a safe range and normal eating has resumed, you can then follow the eating and lifestyle plan in this book to achieve the same results in a safe, gradual, and healthy way, so that you can be wholly healthy and slim, rather than slim and half dead from the ill effects. It will be far more rewarding, and if you work through the other resources in this book, you'll achieve far greater results than weight loss alone.

- **Feeling uncomfortable from injecting insulin** – From experience, I've found certain forms of insulin, particularly long-acting insulin, very uncomfortable. Admittedly, it's tempting to just avoid injecting the stuff altogether and get into the cycle of 'diabulimia'. However this only causes even more problems so we need another solution.

  There are many different forms of insulin to test to find out what suits you best and which regimes you should adopt. If you're not happy with your insulin regime, make sure you voice this to your doctor. They should be there for you and willing to help with any medical challenges you may have.

  When I explained to one doctor the challenges I encountered with long-acting insulin, after trying many different types, I was advised to 'just keep with it and make sure I inject' – not much of a solution or appreciation! I had to carefully devise my own regime, unheard of among most healthcare professionals. It continues to work perfectly well for me, despite opposition from one particular diabetes nurse, who failed to appreciate and listen to my logic and reasons.

  In other words, it's important to test different options, and if you find what works for you and it's safe, have the confidence to stick with it. Be persistent until you get the outcome you want by always keeping your highest intention in mind – to feel comfortable, good, happy, and healthy, without having to avoid injecting altogether.

Generally, when one healthcare professional disagrees and is incapable of helping to find useful solutions, another will agree and be helpful, so keep pushing to get the right help and support that you need. The best answer is always out there; we just have to look a little harder at certain times. Never let this be a reason to resort to dia-bulimia, because it's just as uncomfortable – another paradox, as it seriously intensifies ill feelings, leaving you feeling far worse in many respects. The consultants I choose to work with accept and happily support what works best for me. Anyone who has a problem with something that helps you, when it causes no other problems, isn't in a position or level of thinking to help, anyway, so consulting them is just a waste of time and energy. Avoid practitioners like these, and get the right support for you! I've come across a few too many unhelpful healthcare professionals. You can usually spot them, because they can't seem to manage their own state, never mind yours or mine.

Be sure to keep working with the right people; we all need support, and the right support makes all the difference. Find what works well for you, and get your focus in the right direction. Work on any emotional releases necessary, as well as your personal awareness of what's happening and what needs to happen for you to reach your solution, and you'll get there!

If you first achieve full health and a clear head, you can easily achieve the results you really want in a different way. For example, once you've carefully stabilized yourself and let go of any dia-bulimia traits, work through this book to do the emotional release work, maintain an exceptional mind-set (Chapter Four), and apply the practical steps in terms of diet and lifestyle (Chapter Six). You'll naturally need to reduce your insulin in a safe way, achieving exciting results and healthy weight loss, without any of the gory and deadly effects that dia-bulimia traits bring about.

In my professional work, I always find it touching when I see and hear a person so happy when they've found an alternative way to get what they want. I currently see one person who is now injecting the same small dose of insulin as when she was suffering from dia-bulimia, which is not many units at all! The difference is that she has achieved this safely and is now in full health and great shape, with bags of energy; her life has turned around. So just think what you can achieve!

Hormones and Diabetes

Hormones can get pretty complicated at times, as they all interact and affect one another. Simply put, hormones are chemical messengers produced by one part of the body to tell another part how to optimally function and perfectly regulate various bodily systems. It's when we have too much of one hormone or not enough of another, or the body isn't producing any at all, that things go astray. This is especially so when it comes to regulating blood sugar levels exactly how we want them.

For your own reference I have first provided the main important points and definitions of the hormones that play a key role in influencing blood sugar levels.[9] This will help provide a good understanding why there may be times when your sugar levels don't always seem to make sense, and why maintaining a good natural balance of hormones seriously helps with diabetes management.

Oestrogen and Progesterone

It's often the case that sugar levels increase (irrespective of external factors) in conjunction with the female monthly cycle. Although it's not the same for everyone, quite often sugar levels increase a few days before the start of a period. Generally, this is because the hormones involved in menstruation – oestrogen and progesterone – have been linked to insulin resistance.

Oestrogen and progesterone also have many other interactions with other influential hormones that affect blood sugar levels. For example, progesterone is used to produce the stress hormone cortisol (which we already know elevates blood sugar), and too much oestrogen is associated with lower thyroid hormone (known to lower blood sugar). These two hormones are therefore important considerations when controlling glucose levels.

Thyroid Hormone

Too much or too little thyroid hormone affects sugar levels. The thyroid gland is responsible for regulating metabolism – the process of using and storing energy by releasing a chemical called *thyroid hormone*. If we produce too much thyroid hormone, our metabolism speeds up (hyperthyroidism), and if we produce too little our body functions slow down (hypothyroidism).

If we produce too much thyroid hormone (hyperthyroidism) and our metabolism speeds up, this also means the rate at which insulin and other diabetes medications travel through our body also speeds up. This causes blood sugars to rise, because the required medication to regulate blood glucose levels isn't staying in the body long enough to control it and do the job we need it to.

> *IN A NUTSHELL: Too much thyroid hormone (hyperthyroidism/fast metabolism) = higher sugars*

Alternatively, if we produce too little thyroid hormone (hypothyroidism), our metabolism slows down, which means blood glucose levels can decrease because diabetes medication (insulin or tablets) don't pass through the body as quickly as usual, resulting in it being active for longer.

> *IN A NUTSHELL: Too little thyroid hormone (hypothyroidism/slow metabolism) = lower sugar levels*

In addition, the symptoms of too much or too less thyroid hormone also affect diabetes control itself. For example, in hyperthyroidism, symptoms can appear that are similar to those of a diabetes hypo, leading a person to eat something sugary, when in fact, they likely already have high sugar levels, thereby adding to the problem, if blood sugars aren't checked first.

On the other hand, hypothyroidism involves the following symptoms: feelings of fatigue, lethargy, weight gain, and even depression, which don't help with motivation and good diabetes control. High levels of cortisol (from continued stress) are known to initially decrease thyroid hormone; therefore, when thyroid hormone becomes out of balance in diabetes, it can make blood glucose control far more challenging.

Stress (Gluco-Counter-Regulatory) Hormones

Other hormones, such as *epinephrine (adrenaline), cortisol, human growth hormone,* and *glucagon,* also cause blood sugar levels to rise. This is because the adrenal glands release adrenaline and cortisol, which act directly on the liver to promote sugar production (via *glycogenolysis* – the breaking down of *glycogen,* stored sugar in the liver, into glucose to be released into the bloodstream).

Adrenaline also promotes the breakdown and release of fat nutrients that travel to the liver and are converted into sugar and ketones. It's therefore important to control our adrenaline levels as much as possible by minimizing stress, avoiding too much sugar and refined carbohydrates, cutting down on caffeine, alcohol, drugs, nicotine, and ensuring we are getting enough B vitamins and vitamin C (see Chapter Six for diet and lifestyle information that will dramatically help overall).

Cortisol is a steroid hormone also secreted from the cortex or outer wrapping of the adrenal gland. It makes fat and muscle cells resistant to the action of insulin, and enhances the production of glucose by the liver. Under normal circumstances, cortisol counterbalances the action of insulin, so sugar levels don't drop too low. Under stress, or if high-dose synthetic cortisol (prednisone) is given as a medication (sometimes as an injection for muscle pain, due to it being an anti-inflammatory), cortisol levels become elevated, causing insulin resistance and also increasing sugar levels.

Impact of Continued High levels of Stress Hormones on Diabetes

When continued stress, poor diet, excess sugar and refined carbs, caffeine, alcohol, drugs, nicotine, and vitamin B and C deficiencies are maintained for lengthy periods, the body's adrenaline reserves eventually become depleted, and the immune system is weakened, increasing susceptibility to other illnesses – especially with diabetes to manage on top.

When adrenal function is impaired or weak from overuse, this can naturally cause blood sugar levels to drop, which is obviously dangerous if too much insulin is then unknowingly injected. This can also be linked to low blood pressure, low body temperature, and a total feeling of exhaustion. When stress is prolonged, the organs begin to weaken and other health-related problems are highly likely to arise. This will never prove helpful in stopping or reversing diabetes, as our body needs to be fit and healthy first and foremost to engage in this process.

The resources throughout this book, especially in Chapters Five and Six, will help you avoid or repair any potential adrenal exhaustion resulting from overstimulated adrenal glands, as well as help to dramatically improve and reverse diabetes.

Growth Hormone

Growth hormone is released from the pituitary gland in the brain. Like cortisol, growth hormone counterbalances the effect of insulin on muscle and fat cells. High levels of growth hormone lead to insulin resistance, causing blood sugars to rise. Going through stressful periods also increases growth hormone, again leading to elevated sugar levels.

Stress hormones and sugar levels also rise if we've just had a shock or scare. The fight-or-flight response causes our bodies to produce *catecholamines*, the combination of adrenaline and *noradrenaline* designed to protect us from danger.

Glucagon

In addition to those hormones discussed above, we also have *glucagon*, which is made by the *islet cells* (specifically the *alpha cells*) in the pancreas. Glucagon regulates the production of glucose and other fuels, such as *ketones* in the liver. Glucagon helps the liver to produce sugar (unless its action has been suppressed by insulin and *incretin* hormones, as discussed below).

Glucagon signals the liver to turn *glycogen* (stored glucose) back into *glucose* to be released into the bloodstream. This natural process is called *'glycogenolysis'*. This is what happens when we are injected with GlucaGen (The orange hypo kit) in a severe hypo. This is an exogenous version of glucagon and helps release much-needed glucose back into the bloodstream very quickly.

Glucagon is also released overnight and between meals and is important in maintaining the body's sugar and fuel balance. It signals to the liver to break down its starch or glycogen stores, and helps to form new glucose units and ketone units from other substances. It also promotes the breakdown of fat in fat cells.

Glucose counter-regulatory hormones can also add to high sugar levels when they are naturally responding to correct a low blood sugar level, but instead *over*-correct it. This is referred to as a 'Rebound Reaction' or 'Somogyi Reaction'. It's therefore important to be aware of this reaction so that you can anticipate it, keep a check, and counter it if necessary.

Although glucagon is essential in avoiding low sugar levels, it's also important to ensure we balance this hormone just right in order to avoid sugar levels rising too high (especially at meal times, due to a continued release of glucagon in people with diabetes). Using the resources contained in this book and adopting the measures described in Chapter Six will help you achieve this.

GLP-1, GIP, and Amylin Incretin Hormones

The hormones *GLP-1* (*glucagon-like peptide-1*), *GIP* (*glucose-dependent insulinotropic polypeptide*), and *amylin* ordinarily help regulate mealtime insulin.

GLP-1 and GIP are *incretin* hormones, a group of metabolic hormones that stimulate a decrease in blood glucose levels. When released from the gut, they signal the beta cells to increase their insulin secretion and, at the same time, decrease the alpha cells' release of glucagon. GLP-1 also slows down the rate at which food empties from the stomach, and acts on the brain to make us feel full and satisfied.

Amylin is released along with insulin from beta cells. It has much the same effect as GLP-1. It decreases glucagon levels, slows the rate at which food empties from the stomach, and makes our brain feel that we have eaten a full and satisfying meal.

These hormones create a fall in glucagon and decrease the liver's glucose production, which helps to maintain blood sugar levels. The overall effect is to reduce the production of sugar by the liver during a meal to prevent it from getting too high.

Unfortunately, people with diabetes have been found to have subnormal amounts of GIP, and their beta cells don't respond properly to GLP-1. As amylin is also produced by the beta cells, this too is rendered ineffective. This may explain why glucagon levels are not suppressed during a meal, causing sugar levels to continually rise in people with diabetes. However, synthetic versions of GLP-1, and particularly amylin (known as pramlintide), are now available as injections to control post-meal glucagon and blood sugar levels in individuals with Type 1 and Type 2 diabetes.

There are also natural ways you can increase these hormones to create more balance in the body and allow it to function optimally. For example, adopting a lower carbohydrate diet that is rich in fibre will help, as will making suggestions to your unconscious mind at meal times (once you have engaged in the relevant emotional release work, see the Visualization section for a guideline).

Diabetes, blood sugar levels, and hormones are inextricably linked, so it is necessary to carefully balance our hormones and maintain that balance in as natural a way as possible.

What We Can Do to Naturally Regulate Our Hormones

Take a mind-body connection approach to naturally balance hormones. Remember: Our bodies are extremely clever; when our mind-set and emotions are perfectly balanced, so too is our physiology, hormones included. When our hormones are out of balance, to the extent that they are causing us problems beyond what is expected as natural fluctuations, it can often represent life being out of balance in some other way for us. It's therefore important to ask our unconscious mind (the part that runs the body on autopilot):

What has to happen to regulate my life exactly as I need it to be, in order to reflect this physically and perfectly balance my hormones?

Be honest, and take the first answer that enters your head – trust your unconscious mind. Whatever you find this reason to be, work on it in order to do something about the root cause where possible, and use the other techniques discussed below to help with this.

For example, I have a slight natural increase in blood sugar levels in relation to my monthly cycle, but this is barely noticeable apart from the times when life has really thrown a few curveballs for a period of time. Certainly, when I've had a work overload and increased demands to meet, it can be attributed to adrenaline/cortisol overproduction, neither of which help sugar levels, as mentioned above. So an awareness of this, as well as the effect of sleep deprivation, has proved essential for me, so that I can act and keep everything in check.

Although it's sometimes difficult to change things like workload, I can still ensure I take some time to relax and meditate, giving auto-suggestions to my unconscious mind to correct this and support the body in balancing my blood sugars. I can also temporarily inject slightly more insulin, if and when needed.

Other mind-body health root challenges and suggestions related to hormonal, menstrual, generic female, thyroid, or glycaemic control problems can be found in the table in Chapter Eight (page 211).

Diet

Diet is an important tool for supporting natural hormonal balance. In following a balanced, lower-carbohydrate diet to help stabilize blood sugar (avoiding the highs and lows from carbohydrates), we also help stabilize cortisol and thyroid levels, because these hormones are responsive to erratic blood sugar changes (see Chapter Six for nutrition information).

Eating plant foods that are high in natural phytoestrogens, such as soybeans, *unprocessed* soy foods, linseeds, nuts, whole grains, apples, fennel, celery, parsley, and alfalfa (herb) can help increase natural oestrogens in the body. Phytoestrogens are plant compounds that are capable of binding to oestrogen receptors. They offer a natural replacement for the lost oestrogen effect, and may allay uncomfortable symptoms of the menopause or problems with low oestrogen that are causing blood sugar interference.

Reducing the number of animal products you consume (as well as *processed* soy varieties and meat-like substitutes) and increasing fibre-rich plant foods, such as fruits (berries are best, as they are also lower carb), along with vegetables, grains, and legumes, will help PMS and blood sugar problems, too.

Avoiding caffeine and increasing phytoestrogens and vitamin B6 is thought to have a balancing effect when oestrogen levels are high (as is often the case in PMS). Vitamin B6 is found in yams, leafy green vegetables, and legumes. Research has also shown that taking B6 supplements one week prior to and during a period significantly helped with general symptoms.[10]

Studies have shown that chasteberry extract helps normalize female hormone balance and a host of symptoms attributed to this, if taken every morning over several months. [11]

CAUTION: Before taking chasteberry, be sure to read up on it first, or consult your GP, as chasteberry should be avoided if you have a hormone-sensitive condition, such as endometriosis, uterine fibroids, or cancer of the breast, uterus, or ovaries. Chasteberry extract can also affect dopamine levels in the brain, thereby interfering with the efficacy of medications for Parkinson's dis-ease, schizophrenia, and potentially other psychiatric health conditions.

Avoid Phthalates

Phthalates are chemicals found in plastics and a number of items in daily use. They have been found to behave like oestrogen and have been shown to disrupt the body's endocrine system, as well as being linked to low fertility. We are surrounded by oestrogens, as oestrogen-like compounds are found in food, air, and water, plastic residues, medications, and exhaust fumes. A high-fat, high-dairy, low-fibre diet increases the amount of oestrogen in the body, too.

We are also exposed to oestrogens when we take natural and synthetic sex hormones as forms of contraception or hormone replacement therapies, so finding alternatives may make a significant difference.

This continual over-exposure to chemical oestrogens can disrupt the balance of our natural oestrogens and affect the working of other hormones, particularly progesterone, which also affects blood sugar levels. Another challenge with synthetic oestrogens is that they take up and occupy the same receptor sites in our body as natural oestrogen and can therefore block the normal functioning of necessary natural oestrogen. Synthetic hormones are also far more difficult to rid from the body and can convey a different message to what was naturally intended.

If you suspect any hormone imbalance, and it's adversely affecting things, consult your GP and get advice about what can be done and what are the best available natural remedies *for you* to get things balanced.

Manage Stress Levels

A big one to help keep hormones balanced is to manage stress levels. Have an outlet or personal strategy for releasing any appropriate negative emotions and stresses, such as exercising to get it out of your system, having a good cry, keeping extremely busy, house work, distractions, getting away and having some fun, even having a bath or quick shower. Ensure you get a good seven to eight hours' sleep, whenever possible, as this will help prevent adrenaline and cortisol levels from soaring.

It's important to apply all of the above strategies and keep things as natural as possible in terms of balancing hormones and maintaining good sugar levels. When hormones are kept in balance on a regular basis, the rest of the body will be fit and healthy, too, but a balanced mind and lifestyle comes well before either.

Tips for a Quick Recovery, If Feeling Unwell

You'll have no doubt heard, or perhaps experienced, that anything from a vomiting bug, sore throat, or virus to a UTI can land people with diabetes in hospital; however, by using the right mind-set and following a few guidelines, this can easily be avoided. Simple as it may sound, this drill has kept me away from hospital and the doctor's office many times. Never underestimate the power of the health management strategies I list here; as I've tried and tested all of these in some exceptionally tricky situations.

NOTE: If you're ever in doubt and sense something is seriously wrong, please *do* call a doctor or seek medical advice. There are lots of resources to conveniently help with this in the Resources section of this book, including online consultations for advice from a qualified registered physician or where to obtain basic prescriptions safely from registered doctors.

Resourcing at 42,000 Feet

The last time I had to use every personal resource I could muster was when I became ill mid-flight at 42,000 feet elevation, while flying over the borders of Iraq. We were enroute to the United Arab Emirates to deliver two specific training courses separately, so I *had to* be well – not to mention, it was my first time going to The Emirates, and they had particularly high expectations. The pressure was on.

To cut a long, dramatic story short, I was continually sick for several hours since boarding the flight. I had severe all-over body cramps and felt exceptionally nauseous, weak, and exhausted! At the same time I was dehydrating fast, and my sugars were beginning to rise. I felt like death warmed up, but I needed to avoid panicking and talking myself into something, because it wasn't going to help or change matters.

This episode was particularly challenging, as the accompanying feelings and symptoms were taking me back to my late teens, when I was extremely ill, so keeping my mental state was everything. It was also not easy, as there were discussions amongst the cabin crew about an emergency landing and being met by an ambulance!

If I ended up in a hospital, I wouldn't be discharged anytime soon, and I certainly didn't want to be responsible for an emergency landing in Iraq or Iran, given the current situation. I therefore knew I had to use everything I had within me to avoid this and reassure the crew that I was going to be okay. Moreover, I needed to sort myself out ASAP – as even by my standards, I knew things were serious and I had to do everything possible to turn things around.

I asked the crew if the aircraft carried any form of anti-sickness meds – even basic anti-travel sickness pills that might help me keep fluids down. I knew I desperately needed a saline drip, but that wasn't going to happen on board, though I did ask. Anti-sickness pills were, unfortunately, the one thing I forgot to get before leaving home! That was a major positive learning for me, because without them I would not have been able to get the rehydration I needed, and at that altitude I would have been in serious trouble!.

Thankfully, the crew did carry some basic anti-sickness pills on board, and once these began to have some effect, I was able to hold down a few sips of a good rehydration drink with the right salts/ glucose and electrolyte balance that I needed, as well as inject tiny amounts of short-acting insulin every half hour. I watched my sugars carefully, to keep everything balanced and stable so that I could get to where I needed to be. After I began to feel a little better, I asked for some oxygen to help with my nausea and energy levels. I was well enough to take my seat half an hour before landing and to remain steady going through customs. I was happy to have landed in one piece whilst avoiding the drama of any ambulance.

When we eventually got to the hotel, my partner Johnny thankfully found an all-night pharmacy to get some good rehydration salts, and I did a careful balance of these with small frequent doses of short-acting insulin all week whilst training. Effectively, I was doing what they would have done in hospital with IV drips and a 'sliding scale', just with the resources I had to stabilize myself enough to enable me to work on fully getting myself better.

By doing this and keeping a very strong focused mind-set throughout, the training was a great success, and I even enjoyed it, despite it being a challenging week healthwise. However without applying such tips, the outcome would have been terrifyingly different.

Keep Your Focus Positive

Focus on getting better and feeling well. Focus on solutions. What can you do to help? Even the tiniest things can make a big difference.

Expect it to pass, trust yourself, and be as positive and proactive as possible. What will help you instantly? Aspirin, ibuprofen, cold and flu drink, anti-sickness or anti-diarrhoea pills, rehydration salts, anti-acids? Get someone to ask a pharmacist, if you're unsure, or keep a general supply of these basic but helpful meds for acute remedies.

Change Your Injection/Management Routine to Get a Handle On Things

Inject small amounts of short-acting insulin whilst having sips and small bites of basic foods (if you can), or the rehydration salts, depending on what is more appropriate. Avoid rehydration salts if you don't need them and can eat and drink normally instead. Keep monitoring glucose levels to keep them as stable as possible whilst balancing between giving your body what it needs and the smaller but regular doses of insulin you also require.

Inject every 20 minutes to an hour, to get on top of any infection and prevent or treat ketosis. Remember: This is just temporary, until you're back on your feet and can get back to your regular routine (a bit like taking two steps back in order to take a huge leap forward). The priority is to get well safely. Everything else goes on hold!

Eat Small But Frequent Meals of Whatever You Can Manage

Regular diets/regimes are on hold for now! I've always found ready-salted crisps are a great way to ease nausea, as well as the following: ginger tea; small amounts of light bread and butter or toast; plain, buttered jacket potatoes; plain biscuits, and even chicken soup (which is particularly good for colds and sore throats). If you can keep eating a bit of this and that, it will help keep you stable and able to take in some of the nutrients your body needs.

Drink as Regularly as Possible

Drinking either tea or soda water (with a bit of sugar, if needed) is helpful; however, avoid sugary sodas or fruit juices. If you are unable to eat anything or drink much, get some Dioralyte (rehydration sachets) and drink little sips; dehydration and electrolyte imbalance can really play havoc with diabetes! You'll find these in most supermarkets and pharmacies as a remedy for rehydration after suffering from sickness and/or diarrhoea. These are also useful to have in, if you ever engage in excessive exercise causing excess perspiration. Avoiding dehydration is always a major priority!

Rest and Relax, But Keep Your Mind Distracted

Distractions such as watching television, reading a book or magazine, solving puzzles, and listening to positive/uplifting music can really help. I find I feel better if I can manage to have a nice, long bath whilst watching TV on the laptop with any food, drink, and meds I need at hand (as well as a bucket for reassurance at times).

Allow Time, Then Call the Doctor

Allow yourself time to let it pass, then call your doctor, if you think you might need some antibiotics or other specific remedies. At this point, the earlier you can do this the better. Also check out some of the resources in the Resources section at the back of this book that may help.

Consider the Root Cause of Why You Might Be Unwell

If you feel up to it, after stabilizing yourself as much as possible, work out *why* you may be feeling like you do, so that you can think about tackling the root problem.

Could you have been overdoing it? Is this your body demanding that you rest? Have you left it no other option? Are you stressed, anxious, dreading, or fearing something? Are you giving yourself an excuse to avoid something? What negative emotions could you be manifesting that need to be released? If your current illness or pain is a negative emotion, what is it?

For other considerations, review the table in Chapter Eight, where you will also find positive things you can do about it. Remember: Self-awareness is always the key to solving a large part of any problem, as well as how you respond.

Use Mental and Visualization Techniques to Help

If you're in any discomfort, use the Peripheral Vision technique (described in the Stress section of this chapter) to help you to relax and ease any discomfort. Remember: Endorphins (happy chemicals) are the body's natural morphine (pain relief), so a positive mind-set and distraction is always going to help.

If you know what physically needs to happen in your body in order for a specific problem to subside you can strongly visualize this. You could also apply the Body Scan meditation to auto-suggest waves of calm and relaxation throughout your body, instead of the other specific suggestions given. Or apply whichever sensations you feel will help.

I could go on, but then we'd probably have another book, so I'll keep this section simple. Just know: If you apply any or all of the above tips, you'll find they will help and, in some cases, keep you from a hospital admission. Just always be careful to keep a close eye on any changes, and if in doubt, get the specific help you need ASAP from a medical professional. Keeping a calm and positive mind-set will always help.

An Essential Quick Solutions Travel Kit
for Acute Challenges

Anyone who knows me will also know that I always have a pretty big bag with me, which aside from a lot of papers and general junk, always contains my Quick Solutions kit. Basically, this is a little pouch of all things that I personally deem essential to keep on me when out and about, travelling any long distance, or stored at home. Some of these things can really help to provide quick solutions if and when needed.

Having these things on my person and already to hand at home has often proved extremely useful and on occasion kept me going when necessary. It has certainly aided my recovery quickly when I've been unwell, and most importantly, kept me out of hospital.

CAUTION: If you ever have any symptoms or complaints that persist, it's essential to consult your doctor and always read the label carefully of any medications you take.

Anti-emetics (Anti-Sickness Tablets)

You can ask your doctor for general anti-sickness tablets to keep on you, to prevent vomiting and allow you to keep down fluids and avoid dehydration in an emergency situation. Use as necessary.

Alternatively, see the Resources section at the back of this book, where you can find out how to access a safe, online, assessed prescription for Avomine 25mg tablets (promethazine teoclate). These are for preventing general nausea (due to travel sickness and other causes), so they are handy to keep on you.

The GlucaGen Kit (Injection of Glucagon)

A GlucaGen kit is generally used by others when a person with diabetes is unconscious from hypoglycaemia, but it's important to already have one on you for speed. I've used a little bit of glucagon (the orange GlucaGen kit) myself on occasion, at times when I've been alone and unable to consume oral glucose quickly enough, when insulin has still been heavily active in my system, accompanied by sugar levels dropping rapidly and suddenly. Had I not done this, I could have lapsed into unconsciousness and needed medical attention. I found it perked me up in 10 minutes, enabling me to then eat a biscuit (or some carbohydrates) and giving me the time to calmly stabilize myself, as necessary. It is also a good reassurance aid to always have on you.

Insulin/Blood Monitoring Kit/General Urinalysis Reagent Strips

Insulin and a blood-monitoring kit are essential items to maintain control of diabetes. The Urinalysis Reagent Strips can be specifically requested from your doctor or purchased from a pharmacy. I'd recommend getting strips that indicate not only ketones but also nitrates, proteins, glucose, and leukocytes (white blood cells), so that you can get an overall picture of whether or not you might have anything going on if you've been feeling unwell. You can then act as necessary. For example, increased nitrates in the urine can indicate a UTI; increased leukocytes, that you are fighting an infection; and the presence of protein can provide prompt warning signs of early kidney problems.

If you have ketones, then you know it's likely that you have a background infection, or that you're not having enough insulin and need to act accordingly by injecting small but regular amounts of insulin to correct this, as explained above, in Tips for a Quick Recovery if Unwell. However if you feel very unwell, please consult your GP for advice.

Anti-Diarrhoea Capsules (Loperamide Hydrochloride)

You can easily buy anti-diarrhoea capsules from the supermarket or pharmacy (you don't need to buy the expensive brands). This is pretty much for the same reason as above – to avoid dehydration and any potential electrolyte imbalance. They are convenient to have on hand, as they allow you to continue with your regular activities without any problems or inconvenience. Just remember to acknowledge the root cause of being unwell once you are stabilized.

Rehydration Salts

Rehydration salts can be bought from the supermarket or pharmacy in sachet or tablet form. The best ones will say on the packet: 'Scientifically balanced formula of electrolytes, glucose, and minerals.' Be careful to check that those you purchase have the lesser quantity of glucose in them, and only take them if you have actually been dehydrated and unable to eat or drink very much, otherwise they can prove counterproductive.

Antacid/Indigestion Tablets

If you have been ill (especially vomiting), or have had high blood sugar levels from being ill, antacid tablets will provide light relief by neutralizing any acid until you can stabilize things. They will also help with discomfort that may prevent you from sleeping or properly resting – which of course you need to aid full recovery.

Nystatin (Nystan Oral Suspension) or Chlorhexidine Gluconate Mouthwash

Nystatin is a commonly prescribed antifungal medicine used to treat oral, throat, and intestinal thrush. This can be useful to have at home or if travelling, as thrush in the mouth and throat can occur after being ill or from having high sugar levels. If this does occur it can cause more nausea and therefore needs treating quickly to avoid a continued cycle of ill health. If you ask your doctor, they should be happy to prescribe this on occasion, especially if you are travelling, as a preventative measure.Alternatively, it can be useful to keep a specific mouthwash that also treats oral thrush. You will usually find these in a brown bottle at the pharmacy. They can sometimes stain teeth with regular use, so only use if required.

Ibuprofen and Aspirin

The general painkillers ibuprofen and aspirin are useful to have on you for any acute pain that is proving distracting, until you can sort out the root problem. They can also help stabilize certain situations, allowing you to think more clearly and manage your health in the best way possible during times of distress.

Clarnico Mint Creams and Sachets of Sugar

These particular mints are great for two reasons. First, mints are always handy if you feel a bit off, and second, as these are mint fondant creams, they are very good if you need a quick sugar boost.

Sachets of sugar are useful to have on you in case you can't eat for any reason; you can get a glass of water or lukewarm tea, and add the necessary sugar. There have been times when I've been low and unable to stomach anything, so a sweet drink with a straw has been really helpful.

All of the above items have been useful to me at some point, and certain items have made the difference between needing a doctor's appointment or hospital admission, or not. Remember these items are to help with immediate problems so you can quickly feel better and get to work on solving the real root cause.

Increasing Motivation

In order to lose weight, quit smoking, improve our general health, or start exercising, we have to be in the right frame of mind, otherwise the motivation will never be there. As explained earlier in the chapter, an emotional clear-out and good stress control are the first steps in increasing your motivation.

It's essential to have a compelling reason to do something. Therefore, you first need to identify a strong purpose for acting – something that gives you a real outcome and has great meaning for you. In terms of health, for example, you have to make sure being healthy is important enough to you to take real action. This comes down to how you value yourself and your body. Do you value yourself enough to make health a priority? Ultimately, if you're healthy (meaning emotionally as well as physically), you'll live longer. So, is living long and well important to you?

You may not be conscious of your values, and that may be why you behave in certain ways without really understanding why. You can find out more about how to effectively work with your values in Chapter Nine in the section on Getting What You Want. Once you establish your values and how important things are to you, work through any necessary root issues underlying your lack of motivation. *Then*, the following techniques can be applied to increase motivation in an instant.

1. When you imagine yourself doing the task you need motivating for, do you have a picture?

2. Make this picture big, bold, and bright. Really bring it to life. Make it buzz with energy. Give it a glow. Make sure it's positive! Really use all your senses to connect with it and create an association in your mind.

3. Now have it come zooming toward you at 100 mph, and let it consume you! Feel the motivating charge take over your body, as you are now fully immersed in the picture.

4. Have a clear outcome for doing what you're doing. Know why you're doing it. Have a compelling enough reason, and see yourself having achieved this. *See* what you can see, *hear* all the things you can hear, and really *feel* the great feelings of happiness and satisfaction when you've done it! Keep focused on this and everything you *do want!* Remember: What you wholeheartedly focus on and give your attention to, you get. You also become what you practise and believe.

5 You can also stimulate feelings of motivation by *anchoring* this (creating a trigger) and setting it off when you need that extra stimulation. Also if you have any particular music that really motivates you, have it playing whilst you do the following:

- Remember a time you last felt exceptionally motivated, so fired up and excited you were itching to do something.

- With this memory, see what you saw, hear what you heard, and feel those motivating feelings. Use all your senses, using any scents and tastes that are apparent.
- At the height of these feelings, snap your thumb and index finger together to create your anchor.
- Then as soon as these feelings begin to disappear, release your fingers.
- Now you should have created a motivating anchor (trigger) if you have done this in a very compelling way!
- Now test this by snapping your thumb and index finger together. If it was compelling enough, you'll automatically feel motivated. You can then use this as a quick technique when you need to fire up your motivation, as this will help you to get into the right state of mind.

If you apply everything mentioned under this section on Motivation, and you really want something enough, you'll constantly have the motivation to do it!

If not, you might need to look at what will happen if you don't conjure up the motivation to do something, and utilize any fears you might have. For example, if it's about losing weight, you might not want to be fat and die of a heart attack. Play with it to find what really fires you up, as we all have different motivation strategies!

It is extremely important to focus on what we *do want* as opposed to what we *don't want,* but some people are motivated by a stick (the group that is 'away from' what they actually want). Although this particular focus takes a lot more time and energy, some people need the 'negative fear factor' in order to act and be motivated, so in this respect you have to do what works!

Quite simply, we all work differently, so whether you are motivated by a carrot, a stick, or a rocket even, be aware of what works best for you, and play to it, whilst at the same time being mindful of where your general concentration really needs to be in order to get the best results.

A Weight Loss Technique for Problem Foods

This technique can help if you overindulge in a specific type of food or drink and it's stopping you from reaching your goal (good sugar levels or anything else).

Warning Before Beginning

It is really important you wholly want to do this, as it could put you off the particular food or drink for life unless you do the reverse of this process. To check this is what you really deep down want, ask yourself the following question very quickly, and you must answer instantly with the first thing that comes to mind:

> *Is it okay with your unconscious mind to go ahead and make these changes today?*

The answer will give you an indication if you are ready or not. It's also best to get someone else to ask you this question, so they can make sure you're not saying one thing but doing another, such as saying 'Yes' but shaking your head even slightly, as this can indicate you are not really ready! In which case, avoid this technique! Provided you do definitely want to avoid the food or drink, you can do the following:

1. Think of the thing you like but wish you didn't. As you think about how much you like it, do you have a picture of this in your mind?

2. Notice the details of your picture. Is it:

   - Black and white or colour?
   - Near or far to your face and in what direction? (The exact location)
   - Bright or dim?
   - Big or small?
   - Are you seeing this as a photograph, or are you actually experiencing it?
   - Do you notice any noises, feelings, tastes, or smells?

3. Once you've noted this, clear your mind. Notice the shoes you're wearing, or take a look outside for a moment!

4. Now think of something which you absolutely detest. It could be dog poo (*I've never met anyone who loves it, but you never know!*)

5. Once you have this thing you detest (dog poo, smelly cheese, liver, and so on), think about how much you detest it. Do you have a picture?

6. Once again notice all the details of your picture:

   - Black and white or colour?
   - Near or far to your face? In which direction? (The exact location)
   - Bright or dim?
   - Big or small?
   - Is it like a photograph, or are you part of the picture?
   - Do you notice any noises, feelings, tastes, or smells?

7. Now clear the pictures from your mind. Check the weather again!

8. Now move the picture of what you detest into the exact same location and size as the picture you like. (Please refer to the free audio resource example for the best experience of this.)

   Make sure you use your own pictures that you get in your mind. Be specific and graphic!

9. Now move the picture of what you like to the exact location and size of the thing you detest (so you have swapped them around)

10. Lock these pictures into your mind like hearing a heavy prison door slam shut, and go get a glass of water!

This is a very powerful technique when properly applied so please consult the on-line resource for a full detailed demonstration. If you still find this challenging please consult the resource section to find an appropriate NLP practitioner or hypnotherapist.

Now, would you like some of that thing you used to like... How is it different? Imagine a time in the future when you might be tempted to indulge, how do you feel? I think you get the picture, have fun!

A Few Strategies to Ensure Maximum Effect

- Make sure the thing you detest is compelling enough.
- Make sure the item you like and need to change is specific.
- Make sure there is a difference in the above factors between what you like and what you detest before you begin. If there is no difference, you need to find something you detest that is more compelling.

- Be creative with this as you can always change it back.
- Also be aware that the impact of this technique can integrate at different time intervals afterwards. It may even be the case that until you are next confronted with the item, you find it repulsive!

If you apply all these strategies properly, you will change your internal representation of the thing you like into something you are no longer bothered about and it will assist you in avoiding the problem item! This will enable you to get the results you want far more easily.

The Power of Visualization

Visualization is an incredibly powerful technique, and when it is properly understood and applied it has fantastic results. As the mind generally thinks in pictures and uses all our senses to create memory, using strong imagery can engrave positive messages deep into our neurology and effect physical changes. This is primarily because the part of the mind responsible for running and maintaining our body 24/7 on autopilot is unable to recognize the difference between what is real and what is not real, if we visualize something with enough clarity and detail. But this must be very clear and specific, using all our senses.

Through using PET scan technology, it is known that the same parts of the brain are activated whether subjects are vividly imagining something or experiencing the reality of it. The nerve firing and chemical release is so similar, powerful neurotransmitters allow the mind to influence the body in the same way.

If you've ever had a very realistic, vivid dream and woken up either crying, laughing, or perhaps even stimulated, disturbed, or unsettled by it, then you have experienced this. Although it is 'just a dream', it stimulated a physical response because your body believed it to be real and responded accordingly. You may even have had to question if something has *really* happened or not, when you have simply dreamt about it.

Similarly, we can use visualization to assist in the healing process and activate simple physical changes, such as temperature control, lifting our mood, and achieving various goals. This is because if we see something with enough detail and clarity, our minds will instruct our bodies to physically respond accordingly and make the necessary changes.

One particular case, documented in 1971 by Dr. O. Carl Simonton,[12] a radiologist at the University of Texas, involved a 61-year-old man who had been diagnosed with throat cancer. The cancer was very far progressed, as the man could hardly swallow and his weight had dropped to 98 pounds. The man's prognosis was very poor: doctors gave him only a 5 percent chance of survival after treatment and strongly anticipated that he wouldn't respond well to treatment, as he was already so weak.

Dr. Simonton was curious as to whether he could find a psychological approach using visualization to help this patient. He suggested that he visualize his immune system attacking the cancer, sweeping the cancer cells from his body, and replacing them with healthy ones. The patient then went away and applied this visualization at regular intervals throughout the day. Shortly thereafter, the tumour began to shrink, and the patient's response to radiation was almost free of side effects. Two months later, the tumour had completely disappeared!

This is a case of a successful recovery utilizing the power of the mind. This same patient went on to use visualization to get his arthritis to disappear, and remained free of this condition and the cancer during the six-year follow up period, after which he resumed a regular healthy life.

In our professional practice, we have also witnessed clients make amazing recoveries from sinister conditions, even after they have been told by other doctors that they have no hope, as a result of using the visualization techniques and root cause therapy described in this book. The work principally involves exploring the physical root cause behind a condition, and taking this even further to look at the emotional psychological root behind that. This allows us to discover exactly what really needs treating in order to activate and guide a positive physical result.

On both a personal and professional level, I have experienced very exciting results as a result of applying this work to diabetes, as I have noted previously. In my own life, for example, I notice a significant difference in response when I use visualization while injecting, compared with injecting when I am distracted and having to be quick.

When I do visualization and trance work as part of reprogramming my own mind, I find I end up needing far less insulin throughout the day. In addition, the small amount of insulin I do require has far more of a potent effect than if I don't apply it – to the extent that I can eat nice treats (a muffin, frangipane, vanilla slice, or some such treat) without requiring the additional insulin normally required for them, and without this adversely affecting my sugar levels.

Naturally, it takes some practice to get good results, and certainly, I do better trances and visualization at particular times than at others (especially when busy). Nevertheless, it has made a huge difference in my own life.

As Norman Cousins (known for his immense personal and professional success in the field of healing) said: 'The human mind converts ideas and expectations into biochemical realities'[13] and, of course, it is this that makes all the difference in the results we experience.

NOTE: It is extremely important to monitor yourself carefully and make any adjustments to your insulin or medication doses very gradually, in order to stay safe. You may want to work closely with your doctor during this process to help you make any necessary adjustments safely. Regularly do a B.M. test to avoid any unexpected results, and act accordingly.

Improving Blood Sugar Visualization and Mantra

The visualization that follows is based on how our body works naturally to metabolize glucose, so it can help to visualize this happening inside your own body at regular intervals. This is intentionally kept as simple as possible, because our minds need clear and specific instructions and visualization to have the best impact. Once we stimulate the main aspect of what we need to correct (re-stimulate beta cells), everything else will naturally respond accordingly (such as the incretin hormones discussed earlier).

There is no right or wrong way to effectively visualize; it's just how you see and experience things. For example, white blood cells attacking a virus may be represented by snow showers covering and freezing out the virus. It really doesn't matter as long as it is clear and specific for you representing what needs to happen to get your desired results, and using *all* your senses. I tend to see things as they really are but in more symbolic form, and I work on using my feelings to feel various shifts within my body, such as the insulin sucking out the glucose from my red blood cells. The key is to practise and do what you feel is most comfortable and effective for you. So however you visualize the process of glucose metabolism happening naturally inside you is fine.

I visualize this process myself every time I inject. This way, I suggest to my body to do the process naturally, too.

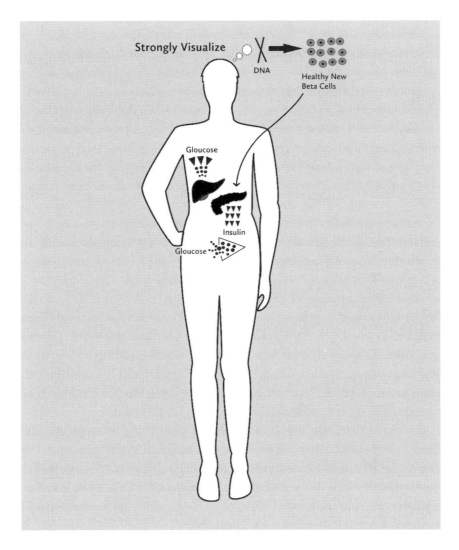

Mantra

Here are the words of an effective mantra that I use while visualizing this process occurring naturally inside me. Based on the work I have done on myself, and with several other people with Type 1, and especially Type 2, diabetes, I can say that this has significantly helped increase the effectiveness of insulin, both reducing the requirement for exogenous (external) insulin and medication and teaching the body how to function normally in the future. Once you warm up and practise this mantra it will become easy, so keep going. You'll also naturally adapt your own shortened version, so just use this one to get the principles to give you the best results.

Unconscious mind, reprogram and stimulate accordingly the other available cells, and deep core ability within my body to function efficiently and rapidly to generate hundreds of thousands of new, healthy, fully functional pancreatic beta cells that I require – beta cells that naturally and automatically secrete insulin and amylin all over my entire nervous system, taking out all the necessary and excess glucose from the red blood cells.

Take it out (actually feeling a pull or suction if you can) easily and effortlessly, storing it in the liver as glycogen to metabolize glucose naturally, continually, and in a safe regular range. You know how to respond accurately to metabolize glucose easily, effortlessly and automatically, as you are making amazing changes in continuing to release diabetes. I can enjoy the sweetness of today, and I am safe. Thank you for your support, positive change, and successful work.

This might sound a little crazy and potentially psycho-spiritual babble at first, but as you know from reading Chapter One and this section, there is a strong science behind this, as well as there being nothing to fear from spiritual connection either. It does, however, require higher level thinking, consciousness, practise, concentration, and being in touch with the part of your mind that runs and maintains your body on autopilot.

I experience significant physical feelings when I apply this mantra using a strong visualization. As I mentioned, the results have been that I've needed far less injected insulin and I have been able to eat treats without requiring any extra units. Along with all of the other work I've done, as documented, this has allowed me to reduce the amount of injected insulin I require and maintain great blood sugar levels.

The nature of this aspect of work is very subjective, so it is best that you experiment with it, practise, and give it some time; patience really is a virtue here! It is necessary to successfully complete all root emotional work before doing this visualization to get the best results.

REMEMBER: The key to the visualizing process is detail, clarity, internal feelings, and repetition. This is what I do *every single time* I inject. The odd times when I am too distracted to successfully visualize, I really notice a difference.

There are other times you can apply this process, too. Here are some of them:

Meditation

This is a useful process to do whilst meditating and making a real internal connection with your mind.

Ultradian Rhythm

Another good time is during a natural biorhythm. This is simply a time when you can naturally access your inner unconscious resources. It's therefore a great time to really use the power of your mind to effectively instruct and communicate with your body. Think of your unconscious as your deepest intuitive attribute.

To do this we can use our natural ultradian rhythm. This is just a natural biological rhythm following a periodic sequence during a 24-hour day. It is when we all naturally go in to a little daydream or a natural trance.

Start recognizing when you have these naturally quiet or 'trance' moments. They usually take place every 90–120 minutes and influence our alertness. During these periods, our unconscious minds are very susceptible and alert, because our conscious mind has drifted – a little like when you've been driving and arrived safely to your destination without even noticing the journey or how you got there.

Natural Sleep Times

Just before we fall asleep or when we are just waking up from sleep are great times to apply any of this work. During such times, effective therapeutic changes can take place. This is because our unconscious mind is responsible for the physiological and psychological occurrences deep within us.

Whenever you find yourself drifting into a natural trance or daydream – a natural state of relaxation – take advantage of it by applying the visualization and language pattern above. Remember: Practise makes perfect, and what you practise and wholeheartedly believe, you become. You see now why I reinforce this so much!

You can also use these moments to make all kinds of positive suggestions, such as those pertaining to general health and well-being, increased energy, calm centredness, or resolve various problems by questioning yourself as discussed in the segment about stress. We all have the answers to the problems we have, it's just a case of whether we are in touch with ourselves enough at that particular time to access them.

If you carefully and fully apply all these resources, you'll experience significant improvements in your blood sugars without increasing insulin or medication, and you will improve your overall physical and psychological health and well-being. For additional support see Resources on page 243.

Remember to be patient and practise warming up to these techniques for the best results. You'll also get the best results by applying the variety of techniques discussed throughout this book, as opposed to just applying one in isolation. The emotional stuff is no doubt the most challenging to overcome, but it is nevertheless crucial to tackle the root manifestation to obtain the results you want.

REMEMBER: No condition is purely physical. The physical cause is merely the symptom of something deeper in our minds, whether we choose to accept it and work with it or not.

When we crack this and really learn to use the power of our minds, the results are unlimited – and the practical work becomes a piece of cake!

CHAPTER FIVE SUMMARY

- Thinking about diabetes differently, more philosophically, is the key to real change.
- When dealing with judgement it helps to be mindful of what is *really* going on. Use your bee suit, and apply the questioning and your inner resources.
- Diabetes burnout provides no solution for anyone; it just worsens any situation.
- Burnout can be avoided and overcome with good awareness and a positive strategy.
- In adopting certain tips, anxiety experienced during a hypo can be greatly reduced.
- Specific techniques and practical strategies assist in powerfully resolving various negative emotions. An audio guide of such can be accessed at www.dr-em.co.uk.
- Meditation has proven, positive health benefits. Body Scan meditation is a great start and reliable method to assist in stopping diabetes and improve general well-being.

- Emotional eating can seriously hinder health when it is out of control.
- Dia-bulimia is catastrophic but can be beaten by applying the right strategies.
- Hormones play a critical role in blood sugar regulation; natural balance is key in this.
- Diabetes can spiral out of control even over minor ailments. Taking certain personal steps to act swiftly can make all the difference for a hassle-free, quick recovery.
- A strong purpose is key to achieving the right motivation. Our motivation is what drives us; the primary reason why we act and get the results we do.
- Visualization is exceptionally powerful because of the way our neurology works.
- Mastering the power of our mind comes down to deep belief and practise.

The Acceleration Plan –
Diet, Lifestyle, Healing Foods, and Complementary Medicine

There are so many additional things we can do to dramatically improve and even reverse diabetes. It all starts with the mind, because a healthy mind equates to a healthy body – and a healthy mind will always be ready to support the body in making significant changes to 'accelerate' this process.

There are already umpteen cookbooks and conflicting dietary advice out there regarding diabetes, so in what I call 'The Acceleration Plan', I have chosen instead to provide a practical guide to assist in stopping diabetes. It incorporates a range of suggestions that, if you follow them, will really make a significant difference and dramatically speed up your result.

When it comes to diet, in this plan, you'll find no pasta, porridge, and rice dishes that would even take a small army all day to burn off. It is a plan that I have developed and that I use myself with great success, meaning it's interesting and sustainable.

When it comes to eating, I'm a big believer in not depriving yourself of something completely (even sugar), unless it's doing you more harm than good. Depriving yourself of a certain food group for any lengthy period of time will only make you want it more, increase the risk of bingeing on it, and potentially result in you missing out on varied nutrients or energy. We still need to keep the body capable of processing food properly. Above all, we want to avoid diet apathy, or a 'mini diet burnout', such as loss of motivation or resentment.

Although this food regime is primarily low carbohydrate (as most carbohydrates are broken down into glucose, and we want to avoid overworking the body), it certainly doesn't deprive you of all carbs. But cutting carbs will also prevent additional sugar cravings, and the less sugar you eat, the less you crave it.

Far less insulin is needed when we follow a lower-carbohydrate diet. But the results go beyond this. I've noticed that those times when I've returned to a regular carbohydrate diet, my insulin needs have been far less than they were the last time I ate more carbohydrate foods. The lower-carbohydrate diet has allowed my body to become accustomed to needing less 'artificial or exogenous' insulin, no matter what I choose to eat. As a result, I now have increased sensitivity to insulin. This is most likely because the lower-carb diet has given my body a rest from needing excess insulin, leading to greater insulin sensitivity when more carbs (thus *slightly* more insulin) were reintroduced.

So the first principle of The Acceleration Plan is that the more the body can adjust to less sugar (in the form of simple and complex carbohydrates), the less it will require injected insulin or medication, and the less over-worked and dependent on artificial support it will be. In effect, this diet assists in retraining the cells in your body, so that they gradually stimulate the desired physical response – able to metabolize glucose independently and easily – as the body has less sugar to process (making the job much easier). This is pretty much like someone having to learn to walk again after a paralysis: it might take some time and dedication, but it can be done with the right commitment and mind-set.

Ultimately, a reduction in the need for external insulin and medication and less natural insulin assists in allowing the body to return to independent functioning. This way, we are helping to reprogramme our bodies and our cell memory. Remember: If you practise something for long enough, you'll eventually know no different. Our cell memory is the same – it needs a good retraining programme!

Evidence of T2 Reversal Using a Similar Diet

There is evidence from various studies that a low-carbohydrate, high-protein, high-fibre diet can stop or reverse Type 2 diabetes. This supports my long-professed belief in the value of this type of diet and offers evidence of efficacy for any cynics. It is also a good platform for under-standing how such a regime can accelerate the process for those with Type 1 diabetes, too.

However, I must emphasize: To sustain long-term successful reversal of diabetes, the main root cause is always emotional; it must be addressed upfront, if you want to accelerate and sustain a wholly successful out-come.

One small study – (Lim EL, Hollingsworth KG, Aribisala BS, Chen MJ, Mathers JC, Taylor R., 2011)[14] proved that Type 2 diabetes can be reversed quickly through dietary changes – in one to eight weeks.

The study was carefully designed to assess the results of a dramatic dietary change on Type 2 diabetes. Volunteers with Type 2 diabetes were asked to consume protein shakes and a low-glycaemic-load, plant-based, low-calorie diet but not to exercise over the eight weeks of the study. After just one week, participants had reversed most features of their diabetes – and all features of their diabetes by the end of eight weeks.

In total, 11 people with diabetes (nine men and two women) were studied and compared with a control group. Through sophisticated techniques, including MRI imaging, they measured the participants' blood sugar and insulin responses, cholesterol levels, and fat in the pancreas and liver (some of the hallmarks of diabetes) before and after dietary changes at one, four, and eight weeks.

What they found was quite astonishing. The beta cells (the pancreas's insulin-producing cells) woke up, and the fat deposits in the pancreas and liver went away. Blood sugars normalized in just one week. Triglycerides dropped by half in one week, and reduced 10-fold in eight weeks. The body's cells became more insulin sensitive and, essentially, in just eight weeks, all evidence of diabetes was gone and the once 'patients with diabetes' looked just like the normal controls on all the testing.

From results like this, it is possible to see the potential effects of this particular diet plan in also dramatically improving Type 1 diabetes by promoting less reliance on exogenous insulin, in addition to other physical and psychological reprogramming, which is key for longevity. But, as mentioned previously, to be successful with this in terms of sustaining long-term complete reversal, it is important to ensure you are also free of long-standing negative emotion. This means addressing the root cause and being aware of this going forward, should any similar root cause situations arise again.

The Lifestyle section of The Acceleration Plan includes general advice for maintaining good overall health that will greatly assist throughout the process of stopping diabetes, both physically and psychologically.

IMPORTANT: When reviewing the advice in the Complementary Medicine section of the plan, please note that at no point in this regime is 'conventional insulin or tablet therapy' completely or abruptly stopped. The

amount of insulin or medication used should only be changed when it be-
comes surplus to requirements and begins to do more harm than good, such
as you find yourself continually experiencing hypoglycaemia.

This does happen, especially as you make the necessary changes to your diet
and lifestyle. In our practice, for example, we've seen continued overmedi-
cation do more harm than good on more than one occasion. Despite this
potential dilemma, you must always consult your physician before making
any such decisions, so that medication reductions can be carefully moni-
tored, and they are made aware of any decisions you make.

Successfully Ditching The Unnecessary

One particular patient we saw in our practice had done so well overcoming serious health challenges that she no longer required a cocktail of
medications for her various mental and physical ailments. However, she
was kept on her medication, because her GP was in denial that changes
of this magnitude could possibly happen. It reached a point where she
was unable to understand why she felt so ill. After we suggested that
she may be taking medication she no longer required, because her old
problems had resolved, she made the decision on her own to function
without the medication. Fortunately, she has never looked back. In
fact, she now works in the emergency services on the front line, doing
a fantastic job – much to her medical team's confusion!

Another study (McGinnis RA, McGrady A, Cox SA, Grower-Dowling KA,
2005)[15] also showed the positive impact of lifestyle intervention on the lives
of those living with Type 2 diabetes.

The study randomly assigned patients with Type 2 diabetes in groups
to receive either 10 sessions of biofeedback and relaxation or three sessions of diabetes education. All sessions were individual, and a total of 39
participants were enrolled, of which 30 completed the three-month study.
HbA1c (average three-monthly blood glucose), forehead muscle tension,
and peripheral skin temperature were measured, and participants were also
scored for depression and anxiety, before and after the study.

This study showed that biofeedback (instrumentally measured awareness of manipulated physiological functions using natural techniques) and
relaxation significantly decreased blood glucose levels and muscle tension,
compared with the control group (those receiving diabetes education). At

the three-month follow-up, the biofeedback group continued to show a decreased blood sugar level and decreased their scores on the depression and anxiety inventories.

Research has also shown that meditation can significantly reduce stress and blood glucose levels, and improve self-care to better manage diabetes. This, in turn, was found to motivate people to exercise more and led to better sugar-level control. Such research shows that making this type of adaptation to an individual's lifestyle has the potential to assist in dramatically improving and stopping diabetes.

Another section in this chapter covers natural supplements, nutrients, herbs, spices and vitamins, all of which can make a significant difference to blood sugar levels.

For example, a study of 60 people with Type 2 diabetes, discussed by naturopathic doctors (Joseph E. Pizzorno and Michael T. Murray, 1999),[16] demonstrated that 1–6 grams of cinnamon taken daily for 40 days reduced fasting blood glucose by 18–29 percent, triglycerides by 23–30 percent, LDL (bad) cholesterol by 7–27 percent, and total cholesterol by 12–26 percent. No changes were found in the control group, who did not take the cinnamon.

Other studies cited in *The Encyclopaedia of Natural Medicine* found that diabetes patients who ate meals with olive oil gained better blood sugar control than those who ate lower-fat meals without olive oil, and that olive leaf extract can decrease blood pressure as well as protect against the oxidation of cholesterol in the blood, thereby helping to prevent heart disease. Such studies suggest how diet and lifestyle can assist in the overall improvement of diabetes and potential or subsequent complications.

Reminder Before Starting

The complementary practices discussed in this section are exceptionally effective and are a fundamental component in helping you to dramatically improve and stop diabetes. However, they do *not* provide a substitute for the gradual and safe reduction of conventional insulin or other prescribed therapy. It is critical that you remain aware of the rapid and powerful effects of lifestyle and nutritional interventions, as you may experience hypoglycaemia unless you adjust insulin dosing accordingly. It's vital to monitor your blood glucose levels regularly and reduce exogenous insulin/medication as needed whilst following The Acceleration Plan. If you remain mindful of this, hyperclycemia will be easily prevented.

The Acceleration Plan: The Diet Basis

IN A NUTSHELL: 50 grams of carbohydrates per day in a high-fibre, varied plant-based diet of vegetables, nuts, seeds, grains, berries, and lean animal protein.

An important principle in this diet is 'everything in moderation', as good balance in nutrition is fundamental to good health. The focus of this regime is to reduce the body's dependency on sugar (carbohydrates – simple and complex) and its need for insulin. This will give the body a rest from its requirement of higher insulin amounts, so that when you do consume more carbohydrates again in the future, the insulin that is necessary will be more effective in the body, and you'll require less of it.

Think of this like drinking alcohol. If a person who drinks regularly (a couple of glasses of wine every night) goes out for a meal and has just one glass of wine, it would highly likely have minimal effect. But if they avoided alcohol for some time, then went out for a meal again and had just one glass of wine, they'd likely feel the effects – perhaps a bit tipsy, relaxed, giddy, or tired. That's because the body has become more sensitive to the alcohol and it takes less alcohol to achieve the same effect.

It's the same principle with insulin – the less insulin you require for a period of time (by refraining from carbohydrates), the less insulin you'll require when you do have carbohydrates again, as the insulin will have a more powerful effect because you'll be more sensitive to it. In this way, you will be training your body to need less insulin (which in turn means less of a compulsion to consume sugar). It means your body will learn to be more self-sufficient, as well as be given chance to regenerate naturally. This also helps with weight reduction, as increased insulin in any individual leads to weight gain.

NOTE: In the information that follows, food options referring to 'From specialist resource – SR' can all be purchased in the UK and Europe through *www.lowcarbmegastore.com* or *www.sugarfreemegastore. com; www.thelowcarbgrocery.com* throughout Canada; *www.locarbconnection.com* throughout the United States; or through other similar stores.

Also, remember it is important to just count 'net' carbs (listed in grams). If the line below the carbohydrate count on food labels list the fibre content of the food, also in grams, you can subtract the amount of fibre (grams) from the total carbohydrate values listed (per serving). Dietary fibre is carbohydrate that cannot be digested, so it does not increase blood sugar levels. If something called 'Polyols' or 'sugar alcohols' is also listed, it is recommended that you can subtract half of this amount in grams from the total carbohydrate count, too. Although some people subtract *all* the polyols, they are still carbohydrates but just have *less* of an impact on blood sugar because they are difficult to digest, so it can be safer to just subtract half this amount than the full amount. Often the 'net' carbohydrates are just listed on food labels; however, if they are not, apply the above. Otherwise you may be over-counting or under-counting carbs!

For further clarification on this, a useful example to look at is shown on the following links. The top link will also provide a list of other sources for low-carb food, if you need to access any, and the second contains very good overall information on diabetes.

http://www.onlylowcarb.com/foodlabels.htm
http://dtc.ucsf.edu/living-with-diabetes/diet-and-nutrition/
understanding-carbohydrates/counting-carbohydrates/
learning-to-read-labels/counting-sugar-alcohols/

PLEASE REMEMBER: The more natural, and unprocessed you can keep your diet, the better all round; you can keep it low cost, too!

Meal Options for Breakfast

- **Bitter melon supplements and soya plant sterol drinks** – These are an essential start to the day, whenever possible, due to their blood-glucose and cholesterol-lowering properties.
- **Low-carbohydrate granola** (clusters of nuts and seeds) – This is nice served with warm or cold milk (lactose-free is best, as the natural sugars are reduced) and a little sugar-free honey, if needed. In the UK, Lizzi's Granola is now available in most large chain supermarkets in different varieties. Good with a handful of berries or natural yoghurt.
- **Natural (plain) set yoghurt** – Try with a small handful of blueberries and a couple of strawberries or raspberries, with an optional sprinkling of low-carbohydrate granola and nuts and seeds mixed with a drizzle of honey.

- **Naturally lower-carbohydrate yoghurts** – The brand Irish Yogurt does a creamy, no-added-sugar yoghurt containing around 7 grams of carbohydrates per serving. Generally speaking, the creamier the yoghurt, the lower the carbs.
- **Grapefruit** – Try it sprinkled with stevia as a sweetener (if desired) or with natural yoghurt.
- **Traditional English breakfast (modified)** – Use good-quality sausage with a high meat content and less filler; bacon or turkey bacon rashers (the latter being the healthier option); Quorn alternative, if vegetarian, but be sure to double-check the carb counts on Quorn replacements – most are okay, but others are not; scrambled or poached eggs; mushrooms; spinach; and tomatoes. Light (low-carb) bread (6–10grams carbohydrate) toasted or fresh (see SR).

  NOTE: Some SR products can be expensive, due to being fresh and having more variety, but if you look carefully in the supermarkets you'll find lower-carb products available. They are not quite as low in carbs, due to the special flour used in SR products. For example, Nimble, Warburtons, and Weight Watchers include some low-carb bread products.
- **Eggs** – Boiled, poached, or scrambled eggs; eggs benedict; frittata; or omelettes with the addition of cheese, spinach, salmon, tuna, mushrooms, onion, pepper, and olive, for example.
- **Scrambled tofu** – Plain or with onions/peppers/mushrooms/olives.
- **Salmon or kippers** – Eat with any of the above options.
- **Rice cakes, oat cakes, or cracker bread** – Eat with cheese and continental meat selection, or salmon slices.
- **Spinach, feta cubes, and mushrooms on a slice of light bread**
- **Low-carbohydrate tortilla wraps** (see SR). To create a breakfast wrap (known as a 'breakfast burrito' in the US), fill a tortilla wrap with any of the above fillings and toast them in a sandwich toaster (this helps to reduce carbohydrates further). These wraps can be used creatively as a great base for many recipes (they are generally high in fibre, flaxseed, and omega 3, too). For instance, you can paste the wraps with garlic and butter and lightly toast them in the oven to make a poppadum substitute or garlic bread replacement. They can even make good substitutes for a thin pizza base or tortillas (if shaped and lightly cooked in the oven) to have with chicken, salsa, chili, or something else). Get creative!

- **Toast** – If you feel like a little toast, use 'light' bread, as explained under 'English Breakfast' above.
- **Lower-carbohydrate breakfast/cereal bars** – Alpen Light is a good natural choice, but there are lots of specific 'low carb' breakfast bar product options available.

NOTE: Any of the above options can be mixed or matched, as long as the carbohydrates are kept to a minimum for maximum results. There is no reason to be hungry on this regime. The mind and body need energy to function – just the right energy!

If you find you are constantly hungry, it may be that you are dehydrated, so make sure you drink 8–10 glasses of water a day; you can count herbal teas in that total.

Lunch and Snack Options

- **Olives and feta cheese, cottage cheese, coleslaw** – Homemade is best (where possible) with boiled/poached eggs.
- **Various omelettes/frittatas** (from low-carb choices) – Have fun with ingredients, and throw in different herbs and spices for flavour.
- **Scrambled eggs with spinach, feta, and mushrooms** – For spice, you could add *falafel* (spiced Middle Eastern ground, deep-fried lentil balls). Depending on the brand, these can be low carb, so just check. Serve with light bread, if desired.
- **Scrambled tofu with mushrooms, basil and pine nuts**
- **Mussels in garlic sauce**
- **Baked courgettes with goat's cheese and mint or other herbs of choice**
- **Salad** – Eat without rice or pasta, and avoid drowning in heavy, sugary salad dressing – a dressing with a mayonnaise and cream base is best or just olive oil and vinegar. Keep the components fresh and natural. For example, you might use rocket (arugula), vine tomatoes, cucumbers, peppers, walnuts, celery, cottage cheese, coleslaw, olives, boiled egg, avocado, mushrooms, onions, and so forth. Be creative. Add your choice of meat, cheese, or fish – either grilled or fresh.
- **Nuts and seeds**– Some nuts and seeds can be quite carbohydrate dense, yet others provide a good snack and health properties, so just check individual nutritional contents on the back.

- **Mini snacks and cheese selections** – These include cream cheese wrapped in salmon, chicken strips, salami sticks, and vegetable sticks (asparagus, cucumber, celery, and so on) to dip in cream cheese, peanut butter, almond butter, or pate. Alternatively use these as toppings for the following: prosciutto ham, salmon, tuna fish, and olives or tofu and hummus.
- **Savoury cracker biscuits** – It's best to check packaging for carb counts, or purchase a low-carb variety. Crackers can have 0.3–3g of carbs per cracker, so just a couple can be a nice addition to a very low carb lunch/snack.
- Oatcakes or lower-carbohydrate rye crispbreads
- Prawn cocktail
- Garlic mushrooms
- **Stuffed peppers** – Made with onions, courgettes, aubergines, or tomatoes with cheese or mince (ground beef), coleslaw, guacamole, mozzarella, and tomatoes.
- **Toasted tortilla wraps (SR)** – Use low-carb fillings, such as warm goat's cheese, tuna, chicken, egg, salmon, and so on.
- **Homemade soups** – It's fun to experiment. Just avoid heavy carbohydrate vegetables and potatoes! Mushroom, onion, broccoli and stilton, chicken, and so on all make tasty and satisfying soups.
- **Warm cooked chicken** – To save time, hot rotisserie chickens are available in many supermarkets. Buy regular roasted or plain, though, unless you need a little boost.
- Baked flan (quiche) without a pastry case (frittata)
- **Burritos** – Make using low-carb wraps (SR). Bake these in the oven to shape and crisp them up, or heated on an iron frying pan or griddle. Fill them with mince, onions, peppers, and mushrooms, and top with grated cheese. Be creative with low-carb ingredients.

Main Meal Options to Keep Things Interesting

- **Any pure cooked meat or fish and accompaniments** – Salmon and yellow fin tuna are particularly a good source of omega 3 oils, with green vegetable accompaniments. Accompany with garlic mushrooms, stuffed peppers, and shredded red cabbage cooked in garlic, and a little low-sugar cranberry juice or a drop of red wine (if desired).
- **Baked camembert cheese (or other soft varieties)** – These work with any of the above. Try asparagus spears to dip in the cheese.

- **Homemade curries** – Mix together meat and various vegetables in a butter chicken sauce or other low-carb curry sauce (the spicier the better, as that often means there is less sugar).
- **Burger stack** – Try a burger topped with melted Swiss cheese or mozzarella, tomatoes, onions, mushrooms, peppers, and asparagus, served with homemade coleslaw, guacamole, garlic mushrooms, and shredded cabbage. You can even use large portobello mushrooms as a substitute for the bread bun, because of the great tough meaty texture. Falafel balls (make sure they are low carb), and olives make great extra side dishes, too.
- **Sausage casserole** – Use good-quality sausage with a high percentage of meat and little filler and plain tinned tomatoes for the sauce (to reduce the sugar content) and add onions and garlic.
- **Leek, or aubergine lasagne** – Leek, and aubergine can substitute for regular pasta in lasagne. Use fresh tomatoes or plain tinned tomatoes for the sauce, and add basil for flavour.
- **Pasta substitute dishes** – You can get creative with vegetables like courgettes by using a 'spiralizer' tool to cut thin strips to act as a replacement for pasta. Alternatively, you can use squash strings as a spaghetti substitute. The taste of spaghetti squash also means you can add all the ingredients you might ordinarily put with a traditional spaghetti dish (which are often naturally low carb). Be careful to avoid overcooking squashes, or they will end up as more of a 'mashed potato' substitute. Although it is good to have variety, it is often better to 'spiralize' low-starch green vegetables like courgettes rather than starchy root vegetables.

  Bake or boil the squash, but if you are in a hurry, you can microwave it. To microwave spaghetti squash, cut it in half lengthwise, and scoop out the seeds. Place the squash flesh side up in a microwave-proof dish, with ¼-cup of water. Cover and cook on high until tender (approx. 10–12 mins,) Once cool, use a fork to scrape out the spaghetti-like strands. Then have fun with different recipes. You can also purchase some good variations of low carb pasta substitutions (SR).
- **Leek cannelloni** – Wrap your filling in leeks rather than pasta or pancakes.
  RECIPE: Simply trim off the leafy tops and roots of the leeks. Then gently but firmly push out the centre layers of the leeks up and out, leaving just the outer tubes. Now you can experi-

ment with the filling. Chop up the inner leek layers, so as not to waste them, and fry in light olive oil with some spinach, chopped peppers, onions, ricotta cheese, or whatever you like to make a nice filling. Then fill the leek tubes with your filling. Often, it's useful to put the filling into a plastic bag and cut the corner of it to pipe more easily into the leeks, if you struggle with this. Now put these into a greased baking dish adding some grated cheddar cheese on the top, and bake until the cheese has melted and it is cooked to your liking.

- **Cabbage Tortillas** – Use cabbage leaves, and you can cut out the low-carb tortillas to make the wraps.
- **Cauliflower or Tofu Risotto** – Use cauliflower as a substitute for rice. You can even fry, roast, or mash cauliflower for some great recipes.
  RECIPE: For a fried rice dish using cauliflower, simply cut the cauliflower into large pieces and grate in a food processor (in short, quick bursts, not blitzing) until it has a rice-like texture. Add some sesame oil to a wok/frying pan over medium heat, and fry some crushed garlic, grated ginger, and any other herbs and spices you like. Then add the cauliflower, stirring it as it cooks until it resembles fried rice. You can then have fun adding any other low-carb ingredients to bulk up this recipe, such as sea food, chicken, or tofu. Just experiment with whatever you like to eat.
- **Using tofu as rice** – Simply chop up the tofu into squares and fry with garlic and olive oil, continually breaking up the tofu as it cooks until it becomes grainy like rice. Cook to your liking, then just add to the dish, as above.
- **Cauliflower Mash** – If you boil cauliflower until soft and mash it with a little butter, you can use this as a substitute for mash potato to accompany certain dishes.
- **Corn beef and tuna hash** – Make a hash or mince with all of the above chopped vegetables. This can be served alone or over tortilla shells made from low-carb wraps baked in the oven and moulded around tin foil balls and sandwiched between another outer layer of tinfoil to hold it in place for approx. 10 mins, until hardened and crispy, to give the right shape.
- **Any meat or fish stir fry** – Cook in olive oil. Water chestnuts and bamboo shoots and French beans are good fillers.

- Chili over tortilla balls – Make this with low-carb wraps.
- Fish pie – Use mashed cauliflower instead of mashed potatoes to make this low carb.
- Spinach, tomatoes, and mozzarella bake topped with poached eggs
- Coq au vin, beef bourguignon, lamb shanks
- Grills – Use good-quality sourced meat. Adapt a traditional English breakfast by adding steak, burgers, chicken, or peppers and onion to make it more of a meal.

Herbs and Spices to Add to Meals or Take as Supplements, If You Choose and Desire

- Garlic
- Turmeric
- Russian tarragon
- Black pepper
- Oregano
- Cinnamon – Cinnamon is a great natural sweetener, too.
- Gymnema sylvestre – This Asian herb is a useful supplement, as it may help to increase the amount of insulin in the body and increase the growth of insulin producing beta cells. It comes in capsules and tea. (More benefits are listed below).

These herbs and spices are listed because they have a specific purpose on this regime. However, all herbs and spices are good to use for flavour in cooking, instead of salt or sugar.

Desserts

- Sugar-free jelly (gelatine/jello) – Jelly comes in various flavours. Serve with single pouring cream and/or whipped double cream and a small handful of berries.
- No-added-sugar or lower-carb yoghurts
- Strawberries and cream
- Eaton Mess – Make this simple but classic English dessert with a shop-bought meringue nest (approx. 12g carbohydrate per serving) filled with raspberries and blackberries mixed with double cream. Make homemade meringue with stevia, if you want to reduce the carb count further, although you could use any artificial sweetener. The more natural ingredients you use, the better.

- **Crème brulee** – This is even better if homemade with reduced natural sugar, but either way, it makes a delicious dessert option.
- **Homemade cheesecake** – Make this at home with less sugar, using low-carb granola as a base.
- **Flapjacks** – These gooey oat bars are best made at home, using low-carb granola and sugar-free honey (this can be purchased from the above SR websites, where desired).
- **Natural set yoghurt with a handful of berries and nuts and a squirt of sugar-free honey**
- **Mini fromage frais yoghurts or mousse pots** – Always double-check the nutritional values of different brands of fromage frais and mousse pots, as the carb and sugar content can vary dramatically. You can find some that have 5–10 carbs per serving.
- **Chocolate éclairs** – Use the frozen variety of chocolate eclairs, as they are quite low in carbs, or alternatively, any cream-filled *choux* pastry bun. Check the package to be sure that the eclairs/pastry bun you choose are low in carbs. Eclairs are usually a better choice for a sweet treat, carbohydrate-wise.
- **Crepes (homemade)** – Fill low-carb tortilla wraps with sugar-free honey or chocolate spread and a few berries, and toast the wrap in the sandwich toaster. Serve with pouring or whipped cream.
- **Shortbread biscuits** – Due to the high butter content, shortbread biscuits tend to be lower in carbs, especially if they are homemade and you can also control the sugar type. Check the package, if shop bought.
- **'No-added-sugar' or 'lower sugar' chocolates and biscuits** – Good choices are available from SR. Dark and milk chocolate 'no-added-sugar' bars are available in certain supermarkets, along with sugar-free marshmallows, boiled sweets, and jellies in the sweet aisle (try a particular orange-branded supermarket in the UK for a good selection). In the US, Russell Stover Net Carb low-carb chocolates and candies are available in most large supermarket chains. Coconut bars, chocolate-peanut bars, and cereal bars with lower carb counts can often be found in the pharmaceutical aisle of supermarkets and pharmacies, near weight-loss products and supplements, and in natural foods stores. New ranges of sugar-free, no-added-sugar, or lower-sugar products can often be found in supermarkets, so it's always worth keeping an eye out for new options.

IMPORTANT NOTE: The more natural the ingredients, the better. Avoid overconsuming sugar-free products, as they can have a laxative effect, which can, in turn, affect electrolyte balance and prove counter-productive. Sugar-free products often contain *'sugar alcohols'* – chemically altered plant carbohydrates – as added sugar substitutes and sweeteners, because they affect blood sugar *less* than starch and sugar. Foods can be 'sugar-free' without being 'carbohydrate-free', so remember to just minus 'half' the content of sugar alcohols as carbs, nevertheless. Sometimes just having a small bit of regular *dark* chocolate (as it naturally contains less sugar) can be a better option to keep things more natural. Everything in moderation is the rule of thumb here!

Drinks and Liquids

The best drink is either still or sparking water with a slice of lemon. It is important to drink at least eight glasses of water per day. Having a glass of water at mealtimes makes this easier, and doing this will also help to detoxify the body and keep you hydrated, thereby maintaining energy levels and good cell and brain function.

- **Bitter melon juice** (for glucose-lowering properties) – This drink is great to have on waking, on an empty stomach (60ml only). As it can taste very bitter, you might prefer to take it as a supplement in the form of capsules.
- **Aloe vera juice** (for proposed improvement to fasting blood glucose) – This is good to drink before bedtime.
- **Lactose-free whole milk, soya milk, or cream**
- **Tea and coffee (decaffeinated were possible)** – Caffeine can deplete nutrients and contribute to restless sleep, so it's good to avoid it whenever possible. Avoid adding sugar to drinks, as this adds up. Use natural sweeteners or cinnamon, if necessary.
- **Herbal varieties of tea, both hot and cold** – If store bought and cold, make sure that the tea does not have any added sugar (many iced teas do, especially in the US). It's best to refrigerate your own herbal teas for a refreshing drink.
- **Ginseng tea** is especially good as it can help lower fasting glucose, A1c, and post-prandial blood glucose levels. It is also possible to get the Asian herb Gymnema Sylvestre in tea form, which is very beneficial, as discussed earlier.

- **Diet soft drinks** – Diet soft drinks (sodas) are best kept to a minimum to avoid consuming unnecessary amounts of aspartame, an artificial sweetener that studies show is not healthful.
- **Sugar-free cordial or light, no-added-sugar fruit juices**
- **Options brand lower-sugar hot chocolate drinks** – The Options brand has several varieties of lower-sugar hot chocolates available. You could even add squirty cream and sugar-free marshmallows on top for a treat. Note: Avoid buying these drinks from popular coffee shop chains when you are out, as they are very high in sugar.
- **Red wine in moderation on occasion, if desired** – Wines from colder countries, such as England or France, are better choices, as the grapes tend to be less sweet, due to the climate.
- **Spirits** – In moderation, spirits are okay (but not sweet liquors). However, all alcohol is best avoided for overall health and to maximize the absorption of nutrients.
- **Small drinks of soya plant sterol** – As noted earlier, whilst following The Acceleration Plan, it is worth having a soya plant sterol drink in the morning to help reduce bad cholesterol and promote good cholesterol. For a low-carbohydrate option, select a soya (dairy-free) variety, which also comes with its own benefits.

The primary objective of The Acceleration Plan is to retrain the body to require less exogenous (injected) insulin in the most simple, interesting, and convenient way possible. The plan serves as an additional resource in your efforts to dramatically improve diabetes and stop the condition in its tracks!

Pictures and recipes of tasty, quick, and low-carb meal ideas that I cook or eat myself can be found by logging onto *www.dr-em.co.uk*. Please email your own pictures and recipes of any exciting dishes you make yourself, as I would love to see them and as a way of sharing your creative ideas with others.

Takeaway and Eating Out Guide
When Following a Lower-Carb Regime

Quick Lunch

Supermarkets and natural foods markets with delis and soup and salad bars are actually really convenient when it comes to lunch on the go. Visit the salad bar, and pack your bowl with peppers, olives, coleslaw, cheeses, tomatoes, cucumber, feta salad, eggs – all the low-carb options you can get. Be sure to avoid the pasta, potato, and rice dishes, though, or anything low carb but covered in gunky, sugary sauces.

Alternatively, for something nice and hot, get the hot plain chicken or other meat options. You could even get a mini salad to go with it, or a tub of olives and feta, cheese selection, rice cakes, and so on. It can also be useful to carry low-carb tortilla wraps with you, so you can make a wrap on the go.

Generally, good food stores, especially delis and those known for quality/indulgent food, also have useful low-carb lunch items, often pre-packaged to go; the cost can mount, if you get carried away, so be mindful! Look for salmon pieces, prawns, carrot sticks, chicken slices, olives and feta mix, fresh tomatoes and pepper mix, cottage cheese, coleslaw, cheese selections, sardines, and various deli selection meats. These are all good for a nice picnic, or use them as an accompaniment to meat, fish, or veggies such as peppers, courgettes, and large, flat mushrooms cooked on a portable barbecue grill.

Fast Food Burger Bars

Although probably best to avoid for temptation reasons, if you're struggling for time, or you're with your friends, just order the burger without bun or any sweet sauces (mayonnaise is often the best option). Other options that might work can be found on the breakfast menu, and include a breakfast tray with just the egg and meat, minus the muffin and hash browns. If you want to bulk things up, see if you can exchange the french fries for salad, or just order separate items.

Asian Food – Chinese, Cantonese, or Thai

Most of the dishes found on the menu in Asian restaurants work well for this particular regime, but avoid any dishes with sweet and sticky sauces or that feature battered foods, such as sweet-and-sour or Cantonese, kung po, satay, Szechuan, piquant, orange or lemon sauce, and so on.

Anything that is plain meat, seafood, or vegetables in garlic, black-bean, or oyster sauce is good, accompanied by Chinese mushrooms, bamboo shoots, water chestnuts, asparagus, aubergines, onions, bean sprouts, bean curd (tofu), or a side of mixed vegetables or mussels. (Avoid rice and noodles, and replace with the listed accompaniments.) Foo yung (egg dishes) and English omelettes are also good to order.

Shredded duck, stir-fried chopped vegetables, or chopped seafood with lettuce wraps also make a good side dish, starter, or snack. The low-carb wraps can also replace the Chinese thin pancakes; sugar-free plum sauce can be purchased from the Special Resources listed, if desired, or just use a tiny amount for taste purposes, if necessary.

It is also possible to enjoy seaweed as a starter or side dish. Request that it be served without added sugar and salt. Satay chicken sticks (request with minimal sauce) make a good starter, as well as king prawns (stir-fried not battered) or mussels.

Generally, there's plenty on the menu that can be adapted to a reduced-carb regime, and remember a few carbs won't hurt – just keep it to a minimum. Most decent restaurants and takeaways are happy to help.

Indian

Sadly, it's best to avoid Indian food in restaurants whilst you are following a lower-carb regime. Make homemade curries, instead, using low-carb tortilla wraps as a substitute bread or chapatti. However, if you are out in an Indian restaurant (and we all need treats), the spicier curries with vegetables are best, because they aren't as sweet; avoid any bread-type dishes. Most good Indian restaurants are also very accommodating when you request less sugar and salt in a particular dish. Just explain why, and make substitutions wherever you can, such as swapping rice for dishes of vegetables.

Steakhouses

These can be a good option if you avoid the potato choices and exchange for mushrooms, onions, coleslaw, or guacamole. If it is necessary to have potatoes, small boiled potatoes are best.

Carvery

In the UK, a particularly good choice when eating out is carveries, especially as it is now possible to get these items as a takeaway, too. As these tend to be a choice of roast meats and vegetable selections, you can choose to keep your options low carb. Just be disciplined! It's best to avoid the York-shire puddings and potatoes and reduce the amount of root or sweetened vegetables and gravy or sauces that accompany the meat and nonstarchy vegetables.

Watch for hidden additions to vegetable dishes. Ask if the chef has add-ed items like cranberry sauce to the red cabbage, for example, as this can dramatically increase the sugar content and leave you with a nasty surprise later after you *thought* you were eating low carb.

French and Bistro

French restaurants and bistros are some of the best restaurant choices, as many options are naturally low carb and the food is rich and filling. Be care-ful not to combine these rich low-carb foods with the complimentary bread or any tempting potato accompaniments. If you have great self-control, al-low yourself just a little bit to satisfy your taste buds; if not, ask the staff to take it back. Out of sight, out of mind!

Generally speaking, it's possible to eat well at most eateries, if they are flexible enough to substitute certain food items for lower-carb ones. Most restaurants are accommodating (especially, if you mention health reasons). Many offer takeaway options now, which can be convenient and allows you to add your own low-carb extras at home. Sometimes I order a Chinese takeaway, then cook some garlic-sautéed spinach and mushrooms at home to go with it. It bulks up the meal and takes minutes to do. Another tip when eating out is, if there is a salad bar, take advantage of the healthy low-carb options available.

By following the diet plan I've laid out, and all the available options, it's perfectly possible to eat a regular and enjoyable diet when limiting carbohydrate intake without any particular fuss. Just familiarize yourself with the different types of food allowed, and plan ahead. The more crea-tive and flexible you can be with this plan, the easier it is to maintain and prove successful. I devised, followed, tried, and tested everything on this dietary plan myself to make sure that it is viable for everyone to follow, no matter your budget and lifestyle. I have found that it generates some pretty amazing results, so have some fun, get creative, and enjoy the jour-ney. Remember: Your intention is your health, so you can live a great life doing everything you want!

Lifestyle Acceleration

When it comes to lifestyle, it's important that you make some significant changes to your daily routine to ensure success in reaching your goals. It's essential that you incorporate enjoyable forms of activity in your daily routine, as this will help with good maintenance of diabetes and regulate blood sugar level further. Naturally, some people are more active or sporty than others, but it's still possible to achieve the same beneficial results, even if you aren't. I promise you, if I can squeeze it in without a fuss, it's well worth a go.

For instance, integrating a pleasant 20–30 minute walk into your daily schedule will soon cover quite a few miles throughout the week, making a big difference both mentally and physically. Even 15–20 minutes of physical activity each day will make a great difference. The key is to make sure it's enjoyable and can easily fit into your day. Certain activities will be more appropriate than others, depending on time, cost, and personal enjoyment. But there's something that fits you, if you give it some thought. For example, consider:

- Visiting your local health club, swimming, or participating in various fitness classes for that extra stimulation. This is particularly good if you like meeting others and need extra motivation by doing activities in a group. You might even consider getting a personal trainer.
- Enjoying nature by doing outdoors activities, such as walking, running, cycling, climbing, kayaking, and so on. There's nothing easier than walking somewhere (if practically and physically feasible), rather than taking the car or bus. If the surroundings and scenery are nice, the activity seems hardly noticeable.
- Engaging in social fun. Going out clubbing, dancing, paintballing, five-a-side, bowling, skiing, even shopping are all good ways to get and keep active whilst having fun.
- Doing some type of activity whilst watching television. Personally, I find exercise equipment pretty monotonous, so I used to go on a cross-trainer and rowing device whilst watching television, even revising, too, at one point, so I didn't even notice I was burning the calories. You can even incorporate some activity when waking in the morning or before sleeping, such as stretching or sit-ups in bed.

- Increasing playful activity with your kids or pets.
- Engaging in adult activity, especially if you explore the Karma Sutra and other creative activities.
- Doing housework, washing the car, taking the dog out, and so on.
- Finally, studies (Ranganathan VK, 2004)[17] have found that by strongly visualizing activity using all your senses, you can actually stimulate physical responses that are similar to having actually engaged in activity. Perhaps this is something you could integrate into a meditation upon waking.

Whatever you decide, it should always be possible to increase or engage in some form of enjoyable activity every day. Again, the more creative and flexible you can be, the easier it will be to get great results.

It's also important to use exercise as personal reflection time to give us the time and space to think about things other than our day-to-day work or routine. So make use of this time for personal contemplation, too.

Any form of activity generates endorphins, so getting more active in our daily lives will naturally add to our sense of well-being; it will support us in feeling good, refreshed, and less stressed. That last one is particularly important for us. We want to avoid stress at all costs, for all the reasons you know by now!

Additional Lifestyle Boosters

Meditation, contemplation, prayer, relaxation, and looking for ways to incorporate personal time into your day are exceptionally important to your health. It has been proven that meditation actually lowers blood glucose, as well as blood pressure. This in turn greatly assists in preventing any potential diabetes complications.

We all work hard in one way or another, so it's vital to laugh and play often, too. We must avoid, reframe, and regularly let go of negative thoughts, attitudes, and limitations. Refer back to Chapter Five for the resources to help you do this.

Taking the time to appreciate and chew food slowly aids digestion, along with an overall focus on what you are eating, thereby helping fuel the body better. As noted earlier, drinking 8–10 glasses of pure water daily also assists with digestion, hydration, and cell and brain function. A good alternative to water is herbal tea, which can have other useful benefits, see some of the listed recommendations for example.

Deep Breathing

Deep breathing exercises are great to practise daily to oxygenate, energize, and calm the body, thereby helping in the same way as exercise and good diet. Breathe in deeply through your nose to fill your lungs as far as you can, then exhale intensely through your mouth. As you do this, feel the calm and energy flow right through you.

Never Underestimate Great Sleep

Aim for a good 7–8 hours of sleep every night to invigorate and refresh health. Sleep is the body's natural healing time. This is because during deep sleep, the production of growth hormone is at its peak. Aside from maintaining glucose levels during sleep, growth hormone speeds up the absorption of nutrients and amino acids into the cells and aids the healing of tissues throughout the entire nervous system. Growth hormone also stimulates bone marrow, where the immune system cells are born, and these naturally protect us against illness as well as aiding healing.

Melatonin, often called the sleep hormone, is produced by the pineal gland in our brain at dusk to help us get to sleep and then throughout the night while we sleep deeply. This is important because this hormone inhibits tumours from growing, stimulates the immune system, increases antibodies in saliva, prevents viral infections, has antioxidant properties, and enhances the quality of sleep. Sleep is therefore crucial to dramatically improve and stop diabetes.

Studies show the value of maintaining a steady and natural rhythm in sleep patterns. Researchers at the University of Toronto Centre for Sleep and Chronobiology (Moldofsky et al, 1975)[18] reveal important insights into how sleep heals.

Dr. Harvey Moldofsky and his colleagues studied the natural rhythm of sleep by interrupting the sleep of a group of healthy volunteers over several nights. Each time the volunteers entered a deep-sleep phase, the researchers would wake them up. After a few nights of these disruptions, the students developed the classic symptoms of chronic fatigue syndrome (ME) and fibromyalgia.

Dr. Moldofsky also conducted another study examining how the immune system reacts to sleep deprivation. Researchers examined natural killer cells, a component of the immune system that attacks bacteria, viruses, and tumours. During the study, 23 men slept about eight hours for the first four nights. On the fifth night, researchers woke up the men at 3 a.m., giving them four hours less sleep than usual. This one interruption to their sleep pattern caused the activity of the natural killer cells to decrease by more than a quarter the next day.

It is important to note here that general research suggests that just three hours' sleep loss leads to a 50 percent reduction in immune system efficiency. Melatonin reaches its maximum potential about an hour after we fall into a deep sleep, so after this time, the body's repair systems go into full swing. We must capitalize on this to achieve full health, healing, and well-being.

Sleep is essential for tissue and cellular repair, optimum brain function, and for the effective circulation of the blood to carry nutrients and oxygen around the body whilst it is relaxed and receptive. It is also a key time for body cleansing to take place, as the lymphatic system picks up waste from cells and also helps to optimize the immune system – a key factor in achieving maximum success in our ultimate outcome regarding diabetes.

Sleep is therefore a very important lifestyle adaption that supports all the other work we do to improve our health. As so many people do not sleep well on a regular basis, this point really needs to be highlighted.

To get a good night's sleep, the following can help:
- Write a list of anything on your mind to help externalize it and create some head space, whether it is minor or major. You might even write some proposed solutions next to each point, so you can work through these the next day and be able to get to sleep.
- Be aware of any niggles or worries, and take action to resolve them rather than manifest them.
- Avoid an overactive mind. Write lists or discuss your day with someone as a means of letting go of it, as well as write down the next day's plans before settling down. This way, you can avoid thinking about it when you're nodding off.
- Allow time to unwind, de-stress, and switch off before going to bed. Avoid computers, television or radio news, or too much mental stimulation.
- Avoid caffeine and other stimulants; enjoy milky drinks or chamomile tea.
- Sexual activity can also be beneficial in helping to physically relieve daily stresses, allowing for good sleep.

By taking action to minimize stress as much as possible, alongside protecting your emotional well-being, you will always accelerate your success in stopping diabetes. You can enhance your overall lifestyle by adopting the points mentioned in the indestructible mind-set, and applying the various stress-busting and anxiety-release tips in Chapter Five.

To briefly remind you of some particularly useful ones to integrate into your lifestyle, below is a brief recap.

A Quick Emotional Re-Start

Whenever the head is immersed fully in water for a few seconds, it is said to stimulate the amygdala, the emotional centre of the brain. This can therefore prove beneficial in starting or finishing the day refreshed, especially if you just want to leave a particular day behind.

Surround Yourself With People Who Are a Positive Influence

Family, friends, and even professionals in the medical arena, for example. I only choose to work with doctors and other health practitioners who are respectful, willing to constructively help. Respect should always be a two way process!

Knowing Yourself and Mindfulness

Having a great level of mindfulness and awareness of life, others, and your own personal goals greatly helps with maintaining a positive focus. Even saying your goals out loud as positive affirmations on a regular basis can keep you positively attuned.

Be thankful and appreciative of all you *do* have, in terms of love and life. When you are grateful, the universal laws of physics respond accordingly, and you'll suddenly find that more of what you do want is being attracted to you. This will help with positivity and an appreciation of what is really important in life – a different level of thinking. This will help with stress reduction and overall health, both psychologically and physically.

Finally, it is important to incorporate fun into life wherever possible, and take action to change things when necessary. Although there may be periods when things appear challenging, there is always something you can work towards. Just give it the focus, attention, and energy required.

If you apply the above lifestyle adaptations, they will accelerate, assist, and support you in dramatically improving, and stopping, your diabetes, as well as provide an excellent framework for good living and overall health.

Natural Herbs and Supplements
That Can Make a Huge Difference

All foods have specific properties that are beneficial to our health in specific ways; others, not so much: certain foods promote health whilst others hinder it. In this section, I will discuss several key nutritional supplements that can assist in dramatically improving diabetes, as well as help in avoiding and healing certain complications.

For instance, it is known that in most vegetables there are nutrients that can prevent and treat many dis-eases, especially those of a chronic or degenerative nature, such as heart dis-ease, cancer, arthritis, and diabetes. As some of these conditions are also *potential* complications of diabetes, too, this is a very important section.

Vegetables provide the greatest range of nutrients and phytochemicals, especially *fibre* and *carotenes,* hence the dietary suggestions I listed earlier. They are rich in vitamins, minerals, protein, and contain very little fat. Most of the fat is in the form of *essential fatty acids*, good fats that help the body move oxygen through the bloodstream to major organs. Good fats also aid cell membrane development, strength, and function, and are necessary for strong organs and tissues.

Vegetables contain carbohydrates, both starchy and nonstarchy. For the purposes of this regime, starchy carbs will be avoided. Below is a list of those vegetables that are great to eat throughout this process, as well as being particularly beneficial in stopping diabetes.

It's also important to mention here that vegetables are often best eaten raw (where safe), or in their most natural form, in order to get the most nutrients from them. Some of the most beneficial carotenes, such as *lutein* (excellent for eye health), are better absorbed from cooked foods or in the case of peppers and garlic by chopping them in order to break down certain ingredients for greater benefit. It is important not to overcook food, to avoid losing vital nutrients. Lightly steam, bake, and stir-fry vegetables to gain the maximum nutritional benefits from them.

Spinach

Spinach is an amazing vegetable to eat whenever possible! Although many people aren't overly keen on the taste of spinach, it's a vegetable that can be thrown into many recipes and cooked in lots of different ways to make it incredibly tasty. It can be especially nice sautéed in fresh garlic and olive oil.

Just a one cup serving of spinach has only 43 calories, is naturally low in sugar, and has excellent properties that serve many purposes – especially those that benefit this regime.

For example, spinach is an excellent source of vitamins K, B1, B2, B, and E, and is also rich in folic acid, carotenes, manganese, and magnesium; it contains double the iron of most other leafy greens. The nutrients found in spinach help restore energy, increase vitality, and improve the quality of the blood. As an alkaline food, it also helps to regulate body pH, which is important in protecting your immune system and essential for great healing.

Another useful property of spinach is that it contains one of the richest sources of lutein, which is excellent for eye health. Researchers have also found that spinach contains at least 13 different *flavonoid* compounds. These are antioxidants that function as anticancer agents, helping to protect the body from stomach, skin, and breast cancers.

Onions

Onions are a great source of vitamins C, B6, B1, and K, biotin, chromium, folic acid, and dietary fibre. I will discuss in detail later why these nutrients are so pertinent to healing diabetes.

Clinical studies have shown that both onions and onion extracts reduce blood pressure, clot formation, and lipid levels. They have also been shown to reduce blood glucose levels as effectively as the prescription drugs tolbutamide and phenformin, which are often prescribed for Type 2 diabetes. The active agent is believed to be allyl propyl disulphide (APDS).In addition, antioxidant properties resulting from their high flavonoid count may also play a significant role. Although discussed in detail later, flavonoids are a group of plant pigments that exert higher antioxidant activity than traditional antioxidants like vitamin C.

Clinical evidence suggests that APDS in onions competes with insulin (also a disulphide molecule) for break-down sites in the liver, thus increasing the lifespan of insulin (a little like the role of amylin). Other mechanisms, such as increased liver metabolism of glucose and increased insulin secretion, have also been proposed.

Their amazing ability to lower and improve blood glucose levels and help maintain a healthy blood pressure (a potential complication of diabetes) helps recondition the body. Onions are an important food to eat liberally on a diabetes healing diet.

Fresh Garlic

Like onions, garlic is a very useful, common, and tasty addition to meals, but its health benefits go far beyond taste. It is an excellent source of vitamins B6 and C, antioxidants, and allicins – all of which have potent healing effects. For example, allicins may increase the secretion or slow the degradation of insulin, increase enzyme activity, and improve glucose storage ability in the body.

Although there have been few concluding clinical studies using garlic to heal diabetes, there are many other health benefits to consuming garlic. Garlic protects against atherosclerosis and heart dis-ease (potential complications of diabetes). Studies have shown that it decreases LDL (bad) cholesterol whilst increasing HDL (good) cholesterol, due to its sulphide content, which also makes the blood less sticky. Other studies have shown that garlic helps lower blood pressure and protects against certain cancers. It is also a potent natural antibiotic.

Garlic is very easy to add into the meals suggested in the dietary portion of The Acceleration Plan, and it is well worth consuming more of it. Use fresh, chopped, or crushed garlic for the greatest benefits.

Biotin

Biotin is a water-soluble B vitamin (B7) and is involved in the production of energy. It is sometimes referred to as 'vitamin H'. It aids in the metabolism of carbohydrates, fats, and proteins, making it a very useful nutrient to support this treatment plan to recondition the body.

Flavonoids

Flavonoids are found in many fruits and vegetables and are essential nutrients in the diet. Their antioxidant activity is more effective against a broader range of oxidants than traditional antioxidant nutrients like vitamins C and E, beta-carotene, selenium, and zinc.

Flavonoids are responsible for many of the medicinal properties of certain health foods, including juices, herbs, and bee pollen. Fruits and vegetables with a dark blue, red, purple, and black colour are highest in flavonoids, and include blueberries, blackberries, red cabbage, black olives, and beetroot. Flavonoids help protect blood vessels from damage, rupture, or leakage. This is important for those with diabetes, who are particularly susceptible to complications of retinopathy and nerve damage affecting certain organs and bodily functions.

Flavonoids work together with vitamin C in the body to protect cells from damage. Flavonoids have a very important role in helping to prevent complications of diabetes and maintaining overall good health.

Olives and Olive Oil

Another great snack to have on the diet plan and integrate into salads and stir-fries is olives and the oil made from them. Olives contain vitamin E and good fats and have many health benefits. Olive oil guards against the oxidation of cholesterol and helps prevent conditions like atherosclerosis (narrowing and hardening of the arteries), a potential complication of diabetes. One study showed that patients who ate meals with olive oil gained better blood sugar control. They also improved their levels of *triglycerides*, compounds of fat and sugar that increase the risk of heart disease when found in high amounts in the body.

Bell Peppers

Studies have shown that bell peppers protect against cataracts, possibly due to their vitamin C and beta-carotene content. They also contain many flavonoids, which, along with vitamin C, have been shown to reduce the risk of heart attacks and stroke. These conditions can also be potential complications of diabetes, so it is worth protecting against them or eating peppers to aid healing.

Bitter Melon Juice or Capsules

Bitter melon has amazing medicinal properties. It is an excellent source of vitamin C, folic acid, zinc, potassium, and dietary fibre and also contains thiamine, riboflavin, vitamin E, magnesium, and manganese, which will be discussed further below.

For centuries, bitter melon (juice, tea, or capsules) has been used to treat diabetes by healers in the Amazon and the Philippines, and by Ayurvedic doctors in India. It is also effective in treating a host of other conditions, such as colic, wounds, sores, infections, and fevers. In India, the leaves are used to treat haemorrhoids, abdominal discomfort, fever, warm infections, and skin dis-eases (especially scabies), proving very beneficial generally.

Most importantly for those with diabetes, bitter melon exerts an important hypoglycaemic (blood sugar lowering) effect, which has been confirmed by scientific studies of both animals and humans. It contains a compound known as *charantin*, which has been shown to have more effect on blood sugar levels than the prescription drug tolbutamide, routinely prescribed to lower blood glucose in those with Type 2 diabetes. It also contains an insulin-like compound called *polypeptide P*, or 'vegetable insulin'. Clinical trials with patients with diabetes have shown that just 2 fluid ounces or 60 millilitres of bitter melon juice has a significant effect on reducing blood glucose levels.

Bitter melon is an important supplement when it comes to stopping diabetes, as it can significantly help recondition the body to more efficiently reduce blood glucose levels. It can help reduce dependence on conventional therapy whilst the mind and body are going through the healing process.

Bitter melon can sometimes be hard to find. The following sources are reliable and can assist you with what you need:

http://www.healthmonthly.co.uk/products_search.php?
search_string=bitter+melon
http://basicayurveda.co.uk/bitter-gourd-karela-juice.html

NOTE: The juice requires a certain palate and dedication. I have found that either the juice or capsules can be used to obtain the desired effect.

Dietary Fibre

Generally speaking, dietary fibre is the sum of those plant compounds that cannot be digested by the secretions of the human digestive tract. Fibre is an important part of The Acceleration Plan diet because studies have clearly shown that Type 2 diabetes is closely related to inadequate dietary fibre intake. In clinical trials carried out with patients with diabetes, increasing dietary fibre through diet or supplementation has been shown to have a beneficial therapeutic effect.

The reason that dietary fibre is so beneficial for those with diabetes is that it encourages delayed gastric emptying, resulting in reduced postprandial (after meal) blood sugar levels. It increases feelings of satiety (fullness), which prevents excess snacking or bingeing on the wrong kind of foods – those that result in ill health or increased insulin (which defeats the point).

Dietary fibre increases pancreatic secretions, which helps improve the body's ability to metabolize glucose. Fibre helps maintain good health in numerous other ways, but those mentioned are key to supporting the dramatic improvement and reversal of diabetes.

Vitamins

The 'B' Group

Found in abundance in vegetables – a cornerstone of The Acceleration Plan diet outlined in this chapter – B vitamins are water-soluble vitamins that play an important role in cell (and particularly carbohydrate) metabolism and overall health. Every vitamin in the B group offers something important in a diabetes healing diet, which makes them perhaps the most important vitamins to include in your regime.

Thiamine (Vitamin B1)

Thiamine was the first of the B vitamins to be discovered. It functions as part of the enzyme thiamine pyrophosphate, or TPP, which is essential for energy production – specifically, carbohydrate metabolism and nerve cell function. I mentioned earlier that it is important to reduce or preferably avoid alcohol. The reason for this is that alcohol destroys thiamine and causes extensive damage in the brain.

Niacin (Vitamin B3)

Niacin-containing co-enzymes play an important part in energy, fat, and carbohydrate metabolism and the manufacture of many body compounds, such as sex and adrenaline hormones. This is a pretty useful vitamin.

Pantothenic Acid (Vitamin B5)

Pantothenic acid plays a critical role in the conversion of fats and carbohydrate for energy production, as well as the manufacture of adrenal hormones and red blood cells. For this reason, vitamin B5 is considered by many nutritionists to be the 'anti-stress' vitamin, due to its role in adrenal function and cellular metabolism. It is also used to reduce cholesterol and triglyceride levels, which can greatly assist with potential complications in diabetes, too.

Pyridoxine (Vitamin B6)

Pyridoxine is important because it is involved in the formation of body proteins and structural compounds, chemical neurotransmitters in the nervous system, red blood cells, and prostaglandins. As we know from previous chapters, chemical neurotransmitters are critical in all health and healing, as they carry needed messages and physical responses around the body.

B6 is also critical in maintaining hormonal balance and proper immune function. As we know from Chapter Five, hormonal balance is very important in maintaining balanced glucose levels. This is important in the healing process, because we need both a healthy immune system and stable blood sugars to stop diabetes and encourage the reversal process.

Folic Acid or Folate

Folic acid works in tandem with vitamin B12 and is extremely significant in healing diabetes. This is because it is critical for healthy cell growth, which of course is our intention – to stimulate new, healthy cell growth following the release of stored negative emotions. Folic acid also helps maintain the central nervous system and the overall normal growth and development of the human body. Folic acid is, therefore, very important in maintaining good general health. It is also a must if a woman with diabetes is pregnant, as folic acid is critical in the development of the nervous system of the foetus; a lack of folic acid has been linked to birth defects.

Folic acid (along with B12 and betamine) also functions to reduce levels of *homocysteine*, which (in higher than average levels) has been implicated in atherosclerosis because it directly damages the arteries and reduces the integrity of the walls of the blood vessels. Both can *potentially* be a serious complication in diabetes, as discussed previously. (Note: Spinach is extremely beneficial, due to its high folic acid content.)

Vitamin B12

B12 is necessary in very small quantities. A deficiency can result in impaired nerve function and can cause sensations of pins and needles or burning in the feet. As these symptoms can also be a sign of potential complications in diabetes, it's important to ensure a balanced diet to cover having adequate quantities. It is only found in animal products, so vegans must supplement with this vitamin.

The Vitamin 'B' Family Overall

Given the above, it's pretty clear why it's so important to integrate all of the B vitamins into The Acceleration Plan diet discussed earlier. B vitamins are contained in plenty of the listed foods, but if you still feel deficient in any area, speak to your healthcare provider to see if they recommend you take a good-quality multi-B vitamin as nutritional support. However, if you eat the right suggested foods, such supplements shouldn't be necessary.

Vitamin C – Ascorbic Acid

Most of the vegetables listed in The Acceleration Plan diet contain high levels of ascorbic acid (vitamin C), which is essential for overall health and cannot be manufactured by the human body. As well as essential in collagen manufacture for holding our bodies together, vitamin C is needed for wound repair, immune function, and to assist in the production of neurotransmitters. It is an important antioxidant and has all-round benefits.

Vitamin A

All vitamins are important and feature heavily in the recommended foods in The Acceleration Plan diet, but some vitamins are more relevant in treating diabetes through diet and avoiding any potential complications of the condition. For example, leafy green vegetables, such as spinach, kale, and broccoli, as well as carrots and whole milk contain a high concentration of vitamin A, which is involved in maintaining healthy vision and skin. As four kinds of vitamin A–containing compounds on the human retina are involved in the visual process, this is very significant.

Vitamin E

Vitamin E helps maintain healthy skin. This is important in the care of diabetes, because skin breakages and wounds can take longer to heal and be more prone to further infection (only in some instances).

General Summary of Vitamins

The vitamins that are necessary in a healing diabetes diet are almost all in the foods listed in The Acceleration Plan diet. It's vital to have a balanced and varied diet to get maximum benefit. If you don't feel that you are getting enough variety in your diet, and feel deficient in any area, it's a good idea to speak to your physician to see if they recommend taking a high-quality multi-vitamin as insurance. 'High quality' means that the supplement contains 100 percent of the daily requirement (RDA) for each vitamin and mineral. It should be taken only once a day.

A daily multi-vitamin can be of great benefit, if needed. A randomized, double-blind, placebo-controlled trial of 130 people with diabetes at the University of North Carolina School of Medicine (*The Annals of Internal Medicine*, 2003)[19] showed that those who took a multi-vitamin and mineral supplement reported fewer infectious illnesses and fewer days lost from work than those in the placebo group.

This trial demonstrates how a 'multi-vitamin boost' can benefit the general well-being and overall health of people with diabetes. The aim in The Acceleration Plan is never to 'mega-dose' on vitamins but to take the recommended amount of a nutrient to maximize health and encourage healing.

Beneficial Minerals

Minerals assist greatly in the improvement and reversal of diabetes. Again, many of the mentioned minerals are readily available in the vegetables listed in the diet; however, mineral supplements can also be used, where necessary and suggested; please discuss this with your GP.

Magnesium

Along with potassium, magnesium is an extremely important mineral because it is the most predominant mineral within our cells. The function of magnesium is centred on its ability to activate many enzymes. Like potassium, it is also involved in maintaining the electrical charge of cells, especially in the muscles and nerves.

Magnesium is also involved in many cellular functions, including energy production, protein formation, and cellular replication – all important in supporting your goal of stopping diabetes. A lack of magnesium can result in heart attacks by producing a spasm of the coronary arteries, restricting the blood flow and oxygen to the heart. Magnesium also increases the solubility of calcium in the urine, thereby preventing kidney stone formation. This is very important, because all such factors help to minimize the potential for diabetes complications and maintain strong health.

Potassium, Sodium, and Chloride – Electrolytes

These are all important minerals because they are *electrolytes*, mineral salts that conduct electricity when dissolved in water. They function together to maintain water balance and distribution, kidney and adrenal function, acid base balance, muscle and nerve cell function, as well as heart function.

These electrolytes are crucial players in healing diabetes. A balanced diet of leafy green vegetables and well-controlled blood sugar helps maintain the correct electrolyte balance and is vital for maximum success on this treatment plan. A good balance can also be maintained by keeping well hydrated. If you are dehydrated for any reason, it's essential to restore electrolyte balance. Powder sachets such as dioralyte (discussed in Chapter Five, if unwell) can really help in this situation.

Chromium – A Recommended Supplement

Chromium is a 'trace element' and has a 'glucose tolerance factor'. As previously mentioned, the positive effects of reduced blood glucose levels have been shown in studies. Chromium is involved in blood sugar regulation, so too much or too little can have a devastating effect on the nervous system.

Considerable evidence now suggests that chromium levels are a major determinant of insulin sensitivity, in that if chromium levels are too low, blood sugar levels may remain high, due to a lack of sensitivity of the beta cells to produce insulin. Chromium is believed to help cells process insulin more efficiently, by way of insulin sensitivity. Several studies have confirmed the beneficial effect of chromium for people with diabetes.

For example, a double-blind, randomized, placebo-controlled trial of individuals who were considered at high risk of Type 2 diabetes because of their obesity and family history of the condition was carried out at Louisiana State University and the results published in *Diabetes Care.*[20] The trial subjects received 1000 micrograms of chromium picolinate per day or a placebo over a period of eight months. During this time, the chromium-taking subjects showed a significant increase in insulin sensitivity midway through the trial, whereas the placebo group showed no significant changes. As no changes in body weight, abdominal fat, or body mass index were found during this study, it is suggestive of an improvement in insulin sensitivity due to chromium.

The average UK diet contains only 13.6–14.7 micrograms of chromium per day, and according to naturopathic doctors Murray and Pizzorono in *The Encyclopedia of Natural Medicine* (Little Brown, 1999), we need at least 200 micrograms per day for it to have any significant effect on diabetes.

Maintaining adequate chromium levels is vital, especially to the stage in this treatment plan of reconditioning and supporting the beta cells. The Acceleration Plan diet will help elevate chromium levels naturally, through the consumption of green peppers, spinach, carrots, nuts, seeds, and butter, wholemeal wraps, and granola. This diet regime will improve chromium action in the body, because it restricts refined sugars and white flour products as well as encourages exercise; however, in order to meet the full daily requirement, it can be worth taking a chromium picolinate supplement for added support.

Manganese – A Trace Mineral

Manganese functions in many enzyme systems, including those involved in blood sugar control, energy metabolism, and thyroid hormone function. It also contributes to antioxidant activity and helps us stay healthy and free of dis-ease overall. By following the diet plan in this chapter, there is plenty of opportunity to absorb the necessary amounts of manganese to have a beneficial effect. Large amounts of manganese are found in nuts, but it is believed that in the UK at least half the required amount of manganese comes from drinking black tea, which, of course, has its own intrinsic benefits – mentally and physically!

Minerals, In General

Minerals function alongside vitamins as essential components in many metabolic processes, as well as the general structure and maintenance of the body – some of which specifically help in supporting the very rapid and dramatic improvement of diabetes, as explained.

The Significance of Plant Supplements

Much research has been conducted into various plant supplements for their beneficial effects on diabetes. It would appear from such studies that there is much in nature that can remedy, support, and assist equally in correcting dis-ease and chronic conditions. As researchers have noted the various effects, here is a summary of the relevant ones.

Cinnamon

Cinnamon is useful for assisting with lowering blood sugar and has many other benefits. Many of cinnamon's unique healing abilities come from the basic components in the essential oils found in its bark. Cinnamon has many uses. It is a circulatory stimulant, a sedative for smooth muscle, a carminative, a digestant, an anticonvulsant, a diuretic, an antibiotic, and an anti-ulcerative, as well as having a unique ability to reduce blood glucose. It is certainly worth adding to meals as a spice. It also makes a nice sweetener for certain dishes. Using more cinnamon and less sugar in desserts can work well.

Russian Tarragon

Russian tarragon is an extremely useful spice to add to meals such as curries and stews, because it contains essential oil compounds with potent anti-fungal activity. An extract of Russian tarragon called tarralin has been used traditionally in the treatments of diabetes, as it may reduce glucose concentrations. This may work by blocking an enzyme involved in *gluconeogenesis* (the breakdown of proteins in the liver to create glucose) and by improving insulin efficiency. Russian tarragon is therefore a good spice to add when appropriate to assist in this process.

Turmeric

Tumeric is a great anti-inflammatory and helps the body destroy mutated cancer cells so that the cancer cannot spread throughout the body. It can also help reduce and prevent the oxidation of cholesterol, thereby reducing damage to blood vessels and preventing heart attacks and strokes. Turmeric may assist in preventing any potential damage or complications until full reversal is complete.

NOTE: You will need to add black pepper to dishes with turmeric in order to activate its healing benefits.

Aloe Vera

Aloe contains *glucomannan*, a fibre that can reportedly drive down blood sugar and make cells more sensitive to insulin; thus proving very useful.

In one trial (Department of Preventive and Social Medicine, Faculty of Medicine Siriraj Hospital, Mahidol University, 1996),[21] the effect of one tablespoonful of aloe vera juice, twice a day for at least two weeks in patients with diabetes, was investigated. The results showed that blood sugar and triglyceride levels in the treated group fell, although cholesterol levels were not affected. Numerous other studies have tested the effects of aloe vera juice and shown positive results. As no adverse side effects were reported from such trials, there's likely benefit in adding aloe vera juice to the diet to support this treatment plan. Although there are other supplements mentioned that display similar effects to aloe vera, the juice from this sap is now more readily available and therefore easier to drink.

Oregano

Oregano is a useful herb for its important antioxidant activity and ability to inhabit bacteria. This is particularly useful to those on a diabetes healing plan, because the healthier you are, the easier, faster, and more dramatic the improvement in diabetes you will experience due to a stronger immune system.

Black Pepper

Black pepper is one of the most common spice additions to meals, but it is so beneficial, feel free to use it liberally. Not only does black pepper have excellent antioxidant and antibacterial properties but it has been proven to stimulate the breakdown of fat cells. It also dramatically increases the absorption of certain nutrients, such as the all-important B vitamins, selenium, and beta-carotene – all of which assist in the metabolism of carbohydrates and efficient functioning of metabolizing glucose. This helps prevent complications of diabetes. Remember to also add black pepper to turmeric, in order to activate turmeric's beneficial properties.

Gymnema Sylvestre (Supplements)

Gymnema sylvestre, also known as 'miracle fruit' or *gurmari*, can be a useful herb to stop diabetes. Its Hindi name, gurmar, actually means 'destroyer of sugar'. It has long been used in India to treat diabetes, as its compounds are believed to improve blood sugar uptake in the tissues, increase insulin secretion, and generate more beta cells in the pancreas.

Although there has been little research conducted on this herb, a few studies have suggested that it may decrease fasting glucose and HbA1C, lower insulin requirements in Type 1 diabetes, and reduce medication requirements in Type 2 diabetes.

I have tested gymnema sylvestre in supplement form myself and can comment that it may well have assisted me in improving my own results. I experienced no ill effects, nor have I read any during my research, so this supplement may be an excellent additional support. As this herb may assist in generating new beta cells, it could greatly help in the reconditioning process and healing of diabetes.

It is most easily purchased in capsule form from herbalist stores. One resource I have found to be convenient, well priced, and reliable is the following:

http://www.healthmonthly.co.uk/swanson_gymnema_sylvestre_leaf?category_id=0&search_fstring=gymnema+sylvestre

All in all, it can be said that many herbs and spices, vitamins, and vegetables provide positive benefits, but those listed are particularly useful for our intentions here. It's easy to integrate them into the regular diet plan – and well worth it for the taste, nutritional return, and physical results.

A WORD OF CAUTION – The foods listed in this chapter contain important nutrients, but due to added preservatives for longer 'sell by' dates, chemical manufacturing processes (chlorine rinses), poor soil quality, weather, and forced growth, vegetables generally do not contain the levels of nutrients they may once have done (there is also reported to be no difference between fresh and frozen). Eat clean, whole foods, including organically grown fruits and vegetables and meat, eggs, and dairy from free-range animals, to ensure that you are deriving the greatest benefit from your diet and getting all the nutrients listed.

Integrating beneficial foods into your diet makes a great difference in all aspects of health. It's important to remember, though, that it all starts with the right mind-set in terms of how our bodies respond to what we feed them, and even the motivation we have to do so. In the apt words of Dr. Deepak Chopra: 'The human mind is the best pharmacy in the world.' This is certainly something I agree with. Having said that, though, success still relies on excellent emotional health and management in order to get this pharmacy dispensing in the first place! Apply *all* of the resources found throughout this book to ensure powerful results; you have the tools.

CHAPTER SIX SUMMARY

- The Acceleration Plan is a series of diet and lifestyle suggestions that can really enhance the process of stopping diabetes.
- The regime involves keeping carbohydrates lower (50g/day) whilst still remaining interesting and sustainable. The less carbs you eat, the less you'll crave them.
- The basic premise of the diet is to assist in retraining our cells to function independently in metabolizing glucose.
- This is like warming up our body for change, similar to having to learn to walk again.
- At *no* point in this regime is 'conventional insulin or tablet therapy' completely or abruptly stopped until it is found to do more harm than good.
- Always inform your doctor any changes you intend to implement.
- Eating clean, whole, and unprocessed foods where possible will always be of a greater benefit because they are more nutrient dense.

- Although integrating beneficial foods into your diet makes a great difference, it all starts with the right mind-set, especially in terms of how our body responds to this.
- We can also improve diabetes by considering factors such as good-quality sleep, regular activity, various psychological techniques, and specific nutritional additions as discussed.
- The human mind is the best 'pharmacy' in the world; however, it is excellent mind-set and emotional health that gets this 'pharmacy' dispensing in the first place!

Dealing With the 'Negitudes' –
and Some Amazing Mind-Body
Case Studies to Inspire You

WARNING – Before reading this chapter, get your bee suit out! Always remember exactly what this book is about, and wholeheartedly reject any negative content found in these pages! Focus on the humour, all that we can do, and learn from.

Time and time again, diabetes has a tendency to attract a conscious, sub-conscious, and even unconscious (totally out of our awareness) bombardment of suggested negativity. This can range from everyday common insinuations of serious complications to insurance issues, not being trusted to hold a driving licence for longer than a three-year period, even being asked to have a flu jab every year due to being in a 'vulnerable group'.

It's vital that we're aware of these negative insinuations, so that we can actively do something about them and prevent them 'unconsciously' affecting our mind-set. It can sometimes seem easier to accept things without question as part of the way of the world, but the continuous build-up of negative messages can really affect our mind-set, attitudes, and ultimately, our physical health, as we know from Chapter One.

For example, I know many people with diabetes who lack confidence, experience bouts of depression, have a continuous background anxiety or nervous disposition, and feel disadvantaged, overly contentious, hard done to, or even an outright liability or special case. But they tend not to know why this is, and can't seem to find an obvious or immediate reason. Considering all the direct and indirect negative messages people with diabetes get over time (especially when these messages are the norm in society), the various emotions people with diabetes report seem pretty natural. This is why we have to make sure we're aware of negative messages, in order to protect ourselves.

I remember when my partner and I had just bought our first property, and we were advised to take out life insurance. Whilst the process for my partner was simple, and a case of filling in a few forms, at the age of 23, I was flatly refused because I had Type 1 diabetes and had previously been admitted to hospital (the reason for my hospitalization was apparently irrelevant).

At the time, I felt angry and written off, because in my mind, the insurance company was giving off a negative message. Although I was very conscious of this, I still allowed the negative emotions to adversely affect me physically. I wasn't aware of it at the time; however, I did eventually realize that there had been a continuous build-up of negative suggestions about diabetes around that time.

The things we choose to believe and accept into our neurology determine our future and the results we get (mentally and physically), so this chapter is dedicated to helping protect us all from the unfortunate 'Negitudes' – negative attitudes and aspersions cast around diabetes. The purpose of this is to bring about a good, conscious awareness, so that we recognize suggested negativity and stop it from infiltrating our neurology and building up to affect our mental and physical health.

Later in this chapter, I have included some amazing case studies that exemplify why we should 'never say never' or simply accept things, particularly negative suggestions.

What Do I Mean By Negative Suggestion?

This refers to a negative comment, remark, or implication made by someone that results in you developing a concern, belief, or something that negatively affects you either consciously, subconsciously, or totally out of your awareness (meaning something is bothering you but you don't know 'what' or 'why').

There may be no substance to the comment – it may not be the case at all or just not applicable to you. Nevertheless, the comment has led you to believe this to be true, leading you to feel and act accordingly.

If we're unaware of them, negative suggestions can affect us in very unproductive ways. They can become a 'self-fulfilling prophecy', and we get exactly what we have been led to expect and have accepted as our deep core values and belief system.

Example of a negative suggestion:

'I think diabetics have worse complications to manage than people with HIV' (paraphrased from a scene in a British soap opera).

The negative suggestion here is that people with diabetes:

1. Automatically have complications;
2. These complications can be 'worse' to manage than 'HIV' complications (which the character was dramatizing and panicking about);
3. 'Diabetics' refers to people *being* their condition. (Note that the comment did not refer to 'HIVers', but rather 'people with HIV'.)

This flippant comment sends a broader negative message of what people with diabetes experience or should expect to experience.

Think of your mind as being like a sponge that soaks up a lot of information. Inevitably, we will be unaware of certain chunks of information and semi-aware (subconscious) of other information being absorbed. In this respect, the more information we're aware of, the more we can wholeheartedly refute it. This will affect our beliefs, and ultimately, our physical health.

A Negative Installation

Taking a negative suggestion one step further is a 'negative installation' – put simply, a strong command given to your mind that is assumed to be true and is certain to happen. This may be far from the truth, or wholly inappropriate, but you are led to believe it without question.

Examples of negative installations:

- 'I'd rather have HIV than diabetes. Doctor says people can live with the virus, but Type 2 reduces life expectancy by 10 years.' – Dr. Max Pemberton, *The Daily Mail*, 18 April 2014
- 'If you don't take folic acid supplements now you will have a spina bifida baby.' (I was 19 and not pregnant!)
- 'This is going to hurt...' (referring to an injection)
- 'You need the flu jab, or you'll be ill this winter, because diabetes means you have a weak immune system.'

These are all unfortunate, real-life examples from the medical profession. I'm sure you, too, could add plenty of similar examples from your own life.

They are 'installations' because they are directly supposing something as a foregone conclusion. You may easily accept this, and fulfil the command, if you believe it to be true. Alternatively, such comments may leave you feeling depressed, fearful, in unnecessary suggested pain, or needlessly ill. (In my own case, nearly two decades of no flu jab and no flu or winter illness proves the latter negative installation to be complete rubbish. But imagine if I hadn't recognize this at the time and believed the medical professional in a position of authority!)

This is important. Whilst the odd negative comment may be brushed off or not have much impact in terms of wider implications, negativity that constantly infiltrates your mind on different levels and through various media – from the medical establishment, adverts, government bodies, and books to magazines, the internet, forums, charity organizations, TV programmes, and teachers – eventually creates a general negative consensus, opinion, and feeling surrounding diabetes.

Negative beliefs projected in many ways then become a general global belief and, before we know it, the association of 'diabetes and depressing gloom' becomes what developmental biologist Rupert Sheldrake calls a '*morphogenic field*' (a belief that, as more and more people become familiar with it, becomes increasingly widely accepted and fulfilled as reality). We become what we learn to believe.

Here are some personal examples you may well relate to. These are examples where my own beliefs were tried and tested to the limit. If I had not been conscious of this, or had not known how to reject them, they would likely have damaged my mind-set, and ultimately, my physical health. I hope that they help to highlight the importance of this chapter, and provide personal encouragement and awareness to always keep a positive 'can do' approach in managing and stopping diabetes, even when people can really 'test and try' you.

My Worst Ever Negative Installation

As briefly mentioned at the beginning of this book, after just having my eyes checked, I was told by a female opthalmic consultant: 'Why didn't you pick this up earlier? You're going blind now.' And then I was told to go and take a seat in the busy waiting room – and that was that. Eventually, I was told by a nurse that I could leave and I'd receive a letter.

First of all, there was an indirect assumption that I'd done something wrong and hadn't been vigilant (incidentally, I had), so I felt blamed. Most importantly, there was a direct 'negative installation' that I was going blind!

At the time, this negative installation left me feeling furious at the way I was treated and spoken to. I hurried out of the hospital and cried my eyes out in utter shock and disarray in the car. It was only after two days of processing this that I started to think rationally: *Sod this. I'm never going to let this happen. I'm in control of my own mind, my own health, and I'm going to look at everything I can do about it, as well as speak to someone who might actually be able to communicate properly.*

After quickly picking myself up and deciding to reject the severe negativity projected, when I changed my thinking I found that there were plenty of options. In fact, all that happened above really never needed to happen at all!

The point being that it's vitally important to never just accept certain negativity (despite what someone in authority tells you). Focus on what you can do to find everything out that can help the situation regarding all that you want to happen. Although in today's society, we are often expected to believe and accept what we are told at face value – especially by medical professionals and the news – it's imperative to question everything, explore alternatives, and think outside the box. Never say never, or simply give up!

If you think about it, we can't ever know something is impossible, because it can only ever be proved possible. And to those who say, 'Yeah, but it is impossible until it's proved possible', that actually still makes it a 'possibility'. It can't not!

For example, some people (believe it or not) still say to me, 'It's impossible to cure diabetes'. This can't be the case, because it's still a possibility and will always remain so. No one can know it's impossible! Plus, we outright know Type 2 diabetes can be reversed, as well as successful islet transplants that have taken place in Type 1 cases, which is massively encouraging for developing even more possibilities using mind-body medicine. I have an exciting development along these lines that I'll make available at a later date, after a little more experimenting on myself first... A great accelerator!

Very philosophical, I know. But my point is that no one has the right to project their limitations onto others. That results in our neurology then seeing the limitation and believing it. I have plenty of case studies later offering evidence as to why!

Continuing with the theme of mounting negativity surrounding diabetes: We must be aware of something in order to alter our consciousness and reject it. I'm talking here about the issue of complications in diabetes.

The complications of diabetes may be one of the most challenging and potentially depressing aspects of the condition. Unfortunately, this aspect of the dis-ease tends to be the focal point of most physicians from the date of diagnosis. For instance, it's a frequent occurrence to read the following in the first paragraphs of medical texts about the complications of diabetes.

NOTE: Before reading the following statement, drawn from a combination of diabetes medical texts, please reject the content on all levels!

Diabetes remains one of the leading causes of blindness, kidney failure, amputations, and heart disease. The combination of nerve and circulatory damage causes many diabetic men to be impotent, and large vessels are damaged to create the most common lethal complications of diabetes, such as heart attack and stroke.

A further example of how the complications of diabetes can often be negatively embedded in healthcare professionals, as well as patients from an early age, and thus needs addressing, is something I was told recently by a senior physician.

We were discussing diabetes and the common perception many doctors have of the condition. Keeping in mind this particular doctor saw me testing and injecting every time I worked. Knowing full well I'd managed diabetes for a long time, he began discussing the inevitability of complications, as if they were a foregone conclusion! As if that weren't tedious enough, he then began telling me a particularly unbelievable story that actually went through me on so many levels.

The doctor was once working in a children's hospital on a 'diabetic' ward, where he witnessed two young girls with diabetes walking around the ward with blindfolds on – and they weren't playing blind man's bluff! When one of the consultants asked them what they were doing out of bed, they replied, 'Practising being blind for when we're older.'

The senior doctor who was telling me this story didn't seem overly alarmed or bemused by it. I like to think his snigger was more out of embarrassment than amusement of the content. This aside, what really alarmed me was the fact that children with diabetes had somehow assumed the prospect of blindness by way of naturally equating it with diabetes. This means that at some point these children had actually had this programmed into their neurology, as they were apparently not old enough to read books on diabetes.

This begs the question: Who exactly had suggested or even installed this in the children to such an extent that it caused them to practise being blind? There had clearly been no positive education or influencing of these children. What really alarmed me was the fact that people fulfil and become what they deep down believe and expect – often very much out of their conscious awareness... poor kids!

My reaction to this story (similar to yours, I'm sure) was one of bewilderment, disbelief, and shock. I just couldn't believe:

1. The senior doctor's conclusive negative consensus on diabetes, despite knowing I was personally managing T1!
2. How much work I had ahead of me to do something about the way diabetes is seen and treated overall.
3. The complete lack of awareness on so many levels.

This story even gets to my partner, too, so I think it's important here to mention that loved ones of people with diabetes can also get very affected by the negatives. It's imperative that everyone around you learns to wholeheartedly reject the negatives surrounding diabetes. This helps to avoid any projection or consequences of their worry onto you. Never accept it from people. There's plenty to be optimistic about, and plenty more we can do about it!

It's also worth mentioning again here that we can also become the people we surround ourselves with, so if your family or friends are generally negative worriers, talk to them or take yourself out of these surroundings. Negativity breeds, and will affect anyone in a detrimental way, both psychologically and physically.

Although the intention of medical doctors and others is to avoid the complications of diabetes, the way this is often communicated is, unfortunately, in an *'away from'* intention. For example, their general behaviour and focus inevitably involves much scaremongering, focusing on the negative possibilities, and unnecessary fretting. This is in contrast to a *'towards'* intention that focuses on the intended outcome (being fit, healthy, and well), and all that can be done to achieve this.

The 'towards' intention is something I personally believe should always be the directional thinking, so as to provide a positive motivation and the encouragement necessary to maintain optimum blood sugar levels and achieve excellent health. This 'towards' approach helps prevent apathy and depression amongst patients – something statistically, and from my clinical experience, is becoming more prevalent.

Of course, we must be aware of what would happen if things were to slip and not be quickly corrected, but this should never be the focus. Therein lies the problem, it seems. Even if complications do arise, the emphasis tends to be: 'You've got complications and this treatment has to happen', as opposed to: 'Okay, you've developed "x", but let's focus on what we can do to improve and resolve it. Let's explore all the best options for you and look at what you can also do now to help improve the situation.'

Although most medical professionals appreciate what is involved in diabetes and the potential consequences of the condition, they can sometimes express little compassion for people living with the dis-ease. In such instances, their negative comments and attitudes are unconsciously, subconsciously, and even consciously filtering through to their patients, leading them to often feel depressed. This also includes what medics may not necessarily say, but rather believe or think themselves; their projection. Whether this is conscious or not to them, positive or negative, patients will still detect this (particularly on an unconscious level). This explains why you may have left the diabetes clinic, for example, and felt a particular way, without having any hard-core explanation for your sentiments.

The Power of Suggestion

When I was first diagnosed with diabetes, at the age of 10, the nurse who broke the news said to me very sincerely, 'You can lead a perfectly normal and healthy life. We'll get you set up with everything you need.' Consequently, I felt very reassured and positive.

Later during my stay, another nurse spoke with me. She asked if I had any worries, and if I was coping with being in hospital. Well, I certainly had no worries; I'd already experienced an induced hypo, and understood everything I'd been told or asked about. I was making friends on the ward, playing in the outdoor park, T-shirt painting, leaning Take That songs (at the time), and doing a self-initiated project about diabetes to explain it to my friends (lucky them, I know!), so I was happily getting on with things.

However, the nurse started telling me that I would be going on a special holiday with other 'diabetic' children where I would have chance to talk about anything scary or worrying me. Although I pretty much instantly said I didn't want to go on any special holiday, she began telling me it would be good to talk about coping with diabetes and any problems I had because I'd feel very different to my school friends (I'd already seen two of them). So from feeling reassured and positive, I suddenly felt quite down, like I should be worried and scared about something.

Thankfully, the first nurse came back on shift and explained I didn't have to go on any holiday unless I wanted to, and most children with diabetes get on just fine and adapt well with no problems. She said that there's nothing to worry about, and we're always here to help if you need us. Brilliant! That's all I needed to hear, and I felt reassured again.

This highlights how two different attitudes made all the difference to what was projected and how I felt as a child. The second nurse had suggested to me problems that were never problems, and that diabetes was something to worry about. So you can see the power of suggestion here – positive and negative!

The psychological side of diabetes is increasingly overlooked. A specific example of this is when I attended the eye clinic for retinopathy and was asked, 'Do you have diabetes?' Aside from me wanting to say, 'What do *you* think, Sherlock? You have my file in front of you', diabetes was, in fact, the unfortunate reason for me being there at the time (physically at least anyway).

I replied 'Yes', and the nurse got out a big red rubber stamp labelled 'Diabetic' and literally banged it down in the middle of my notes – in case anyone might forget, perhaps; with the intensity he stamped it, I was half-expecting my forehead to be next!

My point here is that I was at the eye clinic after being told that I was going blind by their staff because of diabetes; yet, with no regard for my psychological well-being, this man took out the big red stamp, stamped my notes, and left me feeling pointlessly labelled. Moreover, he had no awareness of what he was doing. All I can say is that it's a good job I wasn't experiencing a hypo, otherwise I'd have thought I really was surrounded by zombies.

I observed that this nurse did the same thing to all the other individuals with diabetes (as the door was wide open, you couldn't miss it). And not only did he do it on my first visit but he did it every time afterwards, too – in case, perhaps, I had forgotten about diabetes during a three-month follow-up period. There was absolutely no medical reason or other intention for him doing this (it was already on the last page of notes that I had diabetes, as well as being on their clinic register).

This 'labelling' continued until I told them I only partially had diabetes, as I was in the middle of reversing it. Then, without flinching, the nurse simply put a question mark on my file, instead! (one up from the stamp, at least, and light entertainment for me). I don't think he'd even have noticed if I had my dog and cat in the room with me – unless, of course, they were 'diabetic' and needed stamping, too!

When I looked around at the other people in the eye clinic, they understandably looked and sounded extremely depressed and despondent. From my personal experience, that will happen unless you go into such situations psychologically armoured with a metaphorical 'bee suit' and a *strong* sense of humour.

The general atmosphere in the clinic was made worse by none of the patients being given anything positive to consider or contemplate. Rather, it was heavily suggested: 'Here are your cards you have been dealt. You're a 'diabetic'. It's expected, and this is what happens.'

You already know my thoughts about the label 'Diabetic', which is a static and definitive word, implying no change; you might as well say, 'Doomed'. What a stupid label, which has stuck around for a long time without anyone giving any thought to its implications. Although it got monotonous, each time the red stamp appeared I explained to the nurse that whilst I may currently have diabetes, this is a condition, not a person. 'My name is Emma, and I'm a person, and I currently have a condition' *not* 'My name is Diabetes, and I am a condition', thanks very much!

This is an overlooked psychological aspect of diabetes that can lead to serious depression and mismanagement of the condition. For example, whether we consciously realize it or not, if a build-up of these negative suggestions and common perceptions become the 'norm', and a person feels written off, they have no incentive to stay positive and make the right choices for optimum health. That's when a vicious cycle of ill health, both mentally and physically, begins, as explained in Chapter One and Chapter Five. It's all so needless.

I could relate many instances of the overlooked psychological dimension of diabetes within a medical setting. Unfortunately, the problem is much wider, and extends to the way 'diabetics' are viewed by the media, friends, family, partners, teachers, work, governmental departments, and many others. It's important that we become more conscious of how society labels people, so we know exactly what it is we need to do something about.

A classic example of how being unaware of other people's false negative perceptions and the wider impact they can have causes problems can be found in the story of a young girl with diabetes who was clinically depressed. This ordinarily happy, full-of-life young girl, who enjoyed school and socializing, suddenly began not wanting to go to school, felt uninterested in most activities, and was experiencing regular bouts of anger. Her mum noticed these changes and brought her to see me.

The young girl knew herself that she didn't feel right but was really unsure as to why. After some time talking with her, it became apparent that the girl's close friends seemed to be gradually distancing themselves from her, leading her to feel isolated and depressed.

When I pointed this out to her, it seemed to hit a nerve. We explored all the logical reasons for her friends' changes in behaviour towards her, such as them being busy with schoolwork, family occasions, sports clubs, various commitments, boyfriends, and so on. She seemed quite sure this wasn't the case. I then explained how to confront the issue and get to the root of it, as we covered at the beginning of the book.

On her return to see me, the girl was quite upset: she had discovered the real reason for her friends acting differently around her and distancing themselves. Instead of including her in their usual social activities, her friends had apparently been going to various parties and a local fun fair. They had decided to make excuses and not invite her along, in case she had a hypo, requiring her friends to call her parents or an ambulance and spoil whatever they were doing (or probably what they shouldn't have been doing!).

This is understandable in one respect. Her friends did not want her to come to harm, and they wanted to evade any responsibility at that age or give their game away, if something were to happen. It also signified a lack of understanding and empathy for the girl's feelings and condition. As a result, an unnecessary series of events was occurring that could have easily been avoided. Although the girl did not know all this consciously, she had nevertheless subconsciously detected that something wasn't right, and there had been a distancing from her friends, which resulted in her depression.

All this, unfortunately, came from negative perception and lack of understanding of managing diabetes, as well as her friends being afraid to confront the issue. Equally, if she had initially communicated with her friends about what can be done to prevent a hypo, or what to do if something were to happen, she could have avoided any problems.

It also signifies how even being unaware of or not confronting certain negative perceptions can affect us physically and psychologically, regardless; in this particular case, depression. It's important to be aware of such possibilities and to educate people about diabetes to prevent such problems escalating or having a negative impact. Failing that, at least an awareness of the problem highlights the need for changing friends to a more mature, intelligent group, as such limited thinking never helps anyone.

From lists of occupations people with diabetes are not permitted to engage in, to regular driving checks and challenges with insurance policies, to generally bizarre and negative perceptions of the condition – there are endless factors that could lead to feelings of isolation and depression or frustration in someone with diabetes. However, the irony is that individuals with diabetes tend to be more cautious, more responsible, and more conscientious than people without the condition, because they have more to monitor.

This may seem like I'm reinforcing the negative aspects of diabetes, but the point is that these are the factors that could be very suggestive of a 'can't do', 'incapable' belief, leading to a negative spiral, if we let it. It's critical that we become aware of the negative messages that can build up unconsciously, and learn exactly what we can do to put a stop to them.

As you become more aware of negative suggestions, you'll notice them everywhere. In fact, just earlier today, I walked past a lady working in the supermarket (which, seriously, couldn't have been any stranger timing) at the point she was telling a customer she knew, 'It was diabetes that killed him. There's nothing you can do once you've got it. That's it. It gets you in the end.' Needless to say, it got worse and was in fact a heart attack that actually killed the person she was referring to! Astonished over the belief system this lady had about diabetes (and it sounded like she had Type 2 herself), I just thought

It's not diabetes that killed anyone; it's the mentality. So much for a lunch *break!* So with all these snippets of negativity around, what do we do about it? How do we reject it? Well to start with:

- Be consciously aware of negativity, and question certain beliefs, rather than accept them.
- Outwardly say, 'I wholeheartedly reject that negitude, recognizing it as laughable', then focus on what you can positively do to ensure full health and happiness ... because you can.

- Learn to humour people and certain beliefs, because they don't have the resources to realize their negative projections or that they have been negatively mass hypnotized by the media (or medical education).
- Remember what people say is actually just their own beliefs in relation to themselves. For example, 'complications' is what they might focus on if they had diabetes, or as a medical doctor, it may be what they have seen before, or read, so this is what their focus is on.

What an individual projects is always more about them than you – again, it comes down to how our neurology works. So you are always in control to *choose* the things you want to pick up and focus on in order to formulate your own *positive* projections and belief system. (Basically, sod the 'negitudes', and let them drown in their own negativity. Give yourself the last laugh.) So on that note:

- Always keep focused on your goal and intention, to the extent you are extremely single-minded about it and nothing is going to ever stop you or get in your way. Know your outcome, and enjoy it!
- Always separate a person's intention from their behaviour. By this, I mean that most people are well intentioned; however, their behaviour doesn't always reflect this, so do your best to find their highest positive intention, appreciate it, but make them aware of the negative repercussions of their behaviour in order to change it.

See the section in Chapter Five on Dealing with Judgement for practical examples. Next, have a go at the following:

- Always have a secret smile. You know that you are far better than any negativity, and you know that rejecting it is protecting your health; it is therefore only a harmful thought process to the person it's coming from. We can't control other people's negative thoughts, but we can control our own and what *we choose* to think.
- Above all else, apply the indestructible mind-set, and do what you can to get the results you want – never mind anyone else.
- Finally, remember to have fun rejecting the negatives. Laugh at them. Make an example of them. And really give the 'negitudes' a run for their money in awareness lessons.

Case Studies That Will Inspire You

Now, on a fantastically positive note, here are some cases that are not only encouraging and inspiring but that offer proof of why we should remain positive and apply all of the above. The only limits to what we can do are those we place on ourselves from our own deep-seated belief system and the limitations cast by others that we choose to believe.

These are numerous cases studies where people have been given a terminal or life-changing prognosis, yet they have discovered other methods of healing and have recovered full health. So although the cases that follow involve serious health matters, initially, the point is that it can be easy to accept and actualize negative information at face value. It's therefore important to have a proactive and positive belief system, and to refuse to accept suggested negativity, as this can prove life defining.

When studying the core scientific principles of mind-body medicine – the fact that every single thought we have affects every single cell in the body – it soon becomes apparent that our outer health and behaviour is only a reflection of our inner thought patterns, irrespective of whether we choose to admit this or not.

In this respect, when we talk about something being 'incurable' or 'inevitable', all this really means is that a particular condition can't be treated or cured by outer means, and we must therefore look deep within ourselves to do this from the inside. If we are able and willing to change the way we think, believe, and act, we can make deep positive changes! So you see why I say there's no reason to ever say, accept, or believe *never*. It serves no purpose with regard to our mind-set and results.

CASE ONE: The Case of a 24-Year-Old Man
Documented by Dr. Deepak Chopra

This particular patient came to mind-body specialist Dr. Deepak Chopra feeling perfectly healthy, but he had been given only 90 days to live by his previous doctor, and he was already 23 days into this prognosis.

The diagnosis had come about by accident, following a routine blood test due to an old sports injury. This patient had been diagnosed with a rare blood disorder, and his blood results showed he had severe anaemia, but he was not even displaying symptoms of tiredness. He was told by his doctor that medicine could do very little for him, other than a bone marrow transplant.

The patient was understandably reluctant to go through with such a major operation, especially as he felt no symptoms. As a consequence, his doctor had told him to get all his affairs in order and to prepare for what they deemed to be inevitable! Soon after his diagnosis, quite interestingly, he began to experience shortness of breath and found himself unable to sleep for the first time since his diagnosis. Understandably, in desperation, this patient researched what he could do to cure himself. He began meditating and sought the assistance of Dr. Chopra on healing via the mind-body connection.

In exploring this case further, Dr. Chopra discovered that this patient led a stressful life, including holding down four jobs whilst in school, pushing himself to the limit to keep ahead of school debts, and the pressure of business school itself (the patient had moved from Iran to study in America). The patient had also been taking large doses of vitamin supplements and anti-ulcer stomach medication to soothe his chronic stomach pain. He had also been self-medicating for a sports injury, and such medication is known to suppress bone marrow.

This patient also mentioned that he had suddenly lost his sister to a rare blood disorder when she was in law school! It became evident that the patient's symptoms were stress-related, and he was imitating what he had seen with his sister, so Deepak began to work on this accordingly. After living in a stress-free environment and applying specific mind-body healing techniques for a period of time, this patient outlived his original prognosis and continues to live a healthy life.

This case is yet another example of how the mind and the body are intimately interrelated. It appears that mental perceptions project onto us physically and that subconscious self-fulfilling prophecies are real, connected to what had happened to this patient's sister when she was in college.

Amazing Reports

A major study of 400 spontaneous remissions of cancer, later interpreted by Elmer and Alyce Green of the Menninger Clinic, found that all patients had one thing in common: Every person had changed their attitudes before their remissions, changing their thinking to being hopeful, courageous, proactive, and positive.

There are many cases where changing to a positive way of thinking has led patients to triumph over medical diagnoses. However, there are also cases where this has not proved so. Negative modes of thinking produce corresponding negative self-fulfilling prophecies and frequently result in unfortunate outcomes.

In two very sad separate cases in our own practice, we experienced the loss of two young cancer sufferers, both who unfortunately came to us very late in their diagnosis.

Both patients had a positive and determined psychology, which dramatically helped in assisting them with natural pain relief, reducing fatigue, relieving nausea, and even regressing pulmonary tumours in one case; however, both patients had a very deep-seated belief that they would die young.

One patient was exactly the age she thought she would be, and the other believed that at least one of her group of three friends would get cancer. She also believed bad things happened to her because of a decision she made in her earlier life. Although we told both patients they could release these negative emotions and life-defining decisions, they both believed they couldn't personally do this, that they were undeserving, and (sadly) both were just grateful for us helping them through the process with a little more time.

This case shows that a negative core belief powerfully creates devastating results as much as a positive mind-set and core beliefs create positive results. In other words, they are a self-fulfilling prophecy. The mystery of the mind and its power to effect changes within the body manifest in different ways.

CASE TWO: A Male Tumour Case
Documented by Dr. Deepak Chopra

This case involves a man who began to experience dizzy spells, vomiting, double vision, loss of balance, and loss of motor co-ordination. Following a CAT scan, he was diagnosed with a brain tumour. A biopsy of the tumour was taken and was found to be deadly, rapid-growing cancer; due the location, it was considered inoperable.

The doctors recommended intense chemotherapy and radiation and predicted that without them the patient would be dead within six months. Such treatment would have severe side effects, worse than the present symptoms, and would induce anxiety and depression, and the prognosis would still not be good for full recovery.

This patient could not accept the reasoning behind undertaking this treatment. Instead, he moved to California, joined a meditation group, and undertook a series of healing diets, engaged in exercise, and practised visualization techniques and other mental approaches. In essence, he worked with his mind to activate the desired healing effect in his body.

The man soon began to feel better, and within six months, his symptoms were almost completely gone. He returned to his hometown and underwent another CAT scan, which showed no traces of cancer and no sign that any had ever been present!

Conventional medicine conveniently put this down to a mix-up in the patient's files. However, in analyzing the man's personal experience and earlier symptoms, and the fact that it was an unusual situation, we may conclude that this patient is yet another example of the true power of the mind-body connection – a frightening notion to some.

CASE THREE: Multiple Personality Disorder in Diabetes Documented by Dr. Tad James[22]

This interesting case involves a female patient with multiple personalities, in which one personality has been found to have diabetes and be insulin-deficient while another personality in the same person has not. The personality with diabetes had dangerously high blood sugar levels, but when she changed personality and an attendant drew her blood, allowing for no time for the blood to filter the sugar out through her kidneys or store in the liver, the lady's sugar levels were perfectly normal.

This case demonstrates how changes in the mind dramatically affect physical response to a health condition: it manifests as symptoms one minute, but not the next. This is yet another example of the mind having infinite possibilities.

CASE FOUR: Optical Differences in Cases of Multiple Personality Disorder Documented by Dr. S. D. Miller[23]

Within this fascinating case, one man's left eye is reported to have turned outwards in one personality after being injured in a fight. However, the condition disappeared in the other personalities, with no physical trace of the injured eye.

Numerous similar vision cases and other cases that report the disappearance of allergies once an individual changes personality are exceptionally exciting. They demonstrate how the mind influences physical changes in the body. This is especially so when conventional medical science states that allergic reactions cannot turn themselves on and off that quickly. It also gives rise to the point that the root cause of any health condition goes far beyond the physical cause. From all such cases, it would be a very simplistic view to see *only* physical roots.

This offers further evidence of why we should never just accept so called 'facts' at face value.

CASE FIVE: Spontaneous Healing of Cancer
Documented by Dr. Steven Rosenburg

Dr. Steven Rosenburg notes a case of a curious instance whereby the spontaneous and unexplained healing of cancer takes place. A man had walked into hospital complaining of overall malaise, excessive tiredness, weight loss, and severe abdominal pain. X-rays revealed that he had a large mass in his stomach, and abdominal surgery was performed immediately.

Whilst in the operating room performing surgery on the man, the surgeon discovered a life-threatening condition: a fist-sized tumour in the patient's stomach, three smaller tumours on his liver, and suspiciously hardened lymph nodes. All of these findings corresponded to advanced cancer. It was later confirmed to be a very aggressive and fast-growing type of cancer; one tumour had already replaced part of his liver. To alleviate the patient's pain, the surgeon removed the largest mass and two-thirds of his stomach, but left the cancers growing in the liver and elsewhere in order to avoid greater risk of killing him whilst operating. It was also doubtful that anymore surgery would help him, as the cancer had spread so far.

This case appeared hopeless, and the patient was expected to pass away in the next few months. However, just five months later, at a follow-up appointment, he was very much alive, had put on 20 pounds, and returned to work. Astonishingly, 12 years later, he was back again for a current condition requiring that his gall bladder be removed. The doctors checked to make sure that 12 years earlier there had been no mistake, and it was the same man who had had lethal cancer and recovered.

In his second operation, the surgeons took the opportunity to examine the man closely to check for cancer, but there were no signs of it. The man had had an untreatable cancer that was expected to have killed him quickly, and he had received no treatment from anyone other than his operation to remove only part of it.

From this case it is evident that, in some way, this man's body had naturally healed his cancer, demonstrating further the power of the mind-body connection.

If we explore the biochemistry of the body, we can soon see how all of the cases discussed are possible and the potential for many more marvellous discoveries – especially full Type 1 diabetes reversal. That may just take a little longer, because it's likely to have manifested within the body for a longer period of time and there's a little more reconditioning to do. But reversing Type 1 diabetes is perfectly possible.

As we know science has proved the body has infinite healing possibilities. Further evidenced from the case studies I have included above, we have a lot to be excited about. Knowing how the mind and body are inextricably linked, we have infinite power to self-heal, given the right mind-set, core belief system, and deep rooted change work. There's no excuse to ever give up; in fact, every reason to be optimistic and pro-active about what we can achieve in mind/body medicine: permanent reversal of any type of diabetes.

The case studies in this chapter should convince you that rejecting negativity is worth it. But if not you'll only ever believe it when you do it yourself. You have nothing to fear or lose, and everything to gain. It's your personal choice.

If you need any further inspiration, read the following stories of triumph over the odds.

Swimmer, Gary Hall Jr.

Olympic swimmer Gary Hall, Jr. is an amazing success and inspiration. In 2000, just one year after he was diagnosed with Type 1 diabetes and was told he would never again be able to compete at an Olympic level, he took home his first individual gold medal in the 50-meter freestyle race at the Olympic Games – a great achievement, which he repeated in 2004. Gary Hall is testament to the power of an indestructible mind-set!

Actress, Halle Berry

A successful actress, Halle Berry has never let her diagnosis of Type 1 diabetes get in her way. She now refers to herself as having Type 2 (like) diabetes, as a result of weaning herself off insulin. She is another inspirational public figure living with diabetes, who demonstrates an incredible mind-set and the power of saying no to the negitudes.

There are amazing people in the world, capable of infinite possibilities. Are you one too? Because you certainly can be.

CHAPTER SEVEN SUMMARY

- Although diabetes can attract mass negativity, there's a lot we can do about this.
- Good awareness is key to avoid adversely affecting our mind-set thus physical health.
- The things we choose to believe and accept into our neurology determine our future and all the results we get.
- We must protect ourselves from all the diabetes 'Negitudes'.
- Our mind is like a sponge that soaks up a lot of information; consciously or otherwise.
- The more negativity we're aware of, the more we can refute it.
- Complications can often be the focal point, so we must change this for better results.
- Loved ones can also feel diabetes negativity. They must reject this, too, so that it avoids rubbing off on you. Always talk to people if you feel this is the case.
- The power of suggestion (positive or negative) has a significant impact on how we can feel and respond (without even being aware of why this maybe so).
- A build-up of negativity can lead to a vicious cycle of ill health.
- We can't control other people's negative thoughts, but we can control our own and what *we choose* to think. Keep these positive and 'toward' your intention.
- Our limitations only arise from our own deep beliefs and others *we choose* to believe.
- The case studies show how our health goes far beyond the physical root.
- People are capable of infinite possibilities; so are you!

Doing Something About Complications –
From Dealing With Them to Getting Rid of Them

When things happen – from random acute illness to potential symptoms and diagnosis of complications – it can be easy to get drawn into focusing on the problems. Frankly, complications *are* depressing, and only make matters worse when you are already managing diabetes. As I've said many times: we have to look towards what we *can do* rather than focus on the negative, and also work to prevent complications to begin with.

I can relate to this, because I've been there, so I'm not for one minute saying it's easy to simply snap your fingers, change focus, and start walking on water. But there comes a point when we have to see things from a different perspective, trust ourselves, and do something positive about it.

I know from my own experience how certain issues and unwanted news tend to crop up when you are living with diabetes – and the emotions that brings up. Even if we know what we need to do, it's still extremely important to express our emotions. For example, I'm brilliant at finishing a tissue box, and although I'm a placid and softly spoken person, I can let go when I need to, as you have doubtless surmised from my storytelling so far!

We want to avoid pent-up emotions, then manifesting them physically, as that's just building up toxins in the body and won't allow you to positively move on in a hurry. So let your feelings out (as safely as possible). Go and hit the punch bag, rip up pillows, scream, shout, cry, run (I did once dive into a freezing cold outdoor swimming pool and swam lengths underwater – it actually helped me calm down, release some energy, and think so much clearer – in the warm Jacuzzi afterwards of course). Release them!

Once you've done this, then begin to focus on everything you *can do*. Wholeheartedly believe it, and get as many people to support you in this as possible. Surround yourself with constructive optimism, know your intended outcome, take the actions necessary, and you will do it!

As you know by now, if we focus on the negativity surrounding certain issues, we'll only find more negativity. Seek and you will find!

This isn't just me saying that either, it's actually a science relating to quantum physics, based on the principle of 'like attracts like'. I'll avoid getting into details here (though if you are interested, you can read up on the 'law of attraction' and more on how to specifically apply it, or watch the DVD of *What the Bleep Do We Know!? Down the Rabbit Hole*).

Focusing positively on everything you do want to attract is so important. You must wholeheartedly, deep down believe this. Imagine living in a "yes" universe whereby whatever you say (and deep down believe to be true;) the universe says yes to you. I appreciate that I probably do go on about this, but it's for a reason. It is critical to your success in improving and reversing diabetes. So many people say they know this, but never do it, and wonder why things are what they are!

To avoid fixating on the negatives of diabetes, which can be so easy to do, I have little mantras, or repeated sayings, that can be used to retune your psychological focus. They ease things, and provide you with positive suggestions on how you might change a specific situation. They work by providing the mind with a pro-active distraction and reprogramming thoughts.

A 'positive mantra', or affirmation, provides a positive thought pattern and 'auto-suggestion' to your conscious and unconscious mind, and by extension, to your body.

Below, you'll find mantras you can use to re-adjust and distract your mind in a positive way, along with the different situations when you might use them. You'll find these thought patterns very useful, if you apply them properly. They focus on the possible root emotional conflicts behind particular complaints, their metaphysical meaning; in other words, the underlying meaning of certain physical complaints, emotionally and psychologically.

If you are in touch with your inner self, you will know what resonates for you, and have a precise awareness of this, so see these thought patterns as a guide to help you discover the emotional root of whatever is going on physically. Remember: Everything that happens to us *physically* represents our *emotional* health in some way.

The great news here is that, once we get a true awareness of the emotional root, we can change it, and begin to change our physical health. It is exciting that we have a proactive, multi-pronged approach to work with diabetes and its potential complications. This has helped me on many occasions.

For example, *after* my diagnosis of retinopathy, I suddenly experienced what seemed like large black blotches of ink roaming back and forth across my eye. As you can imagine, this was immensely distracting, as sometimes I was in practice, in the middle of a training, or just out having fun. It was easy to get into a panic and spiral of worry, leading to a low mood, if I let it – particularly after the 'negative installation' I'd been given by 'Dr. Doom'.

I knew panic would in no way help the situation, nor would getting down about it, and there was nothing I could do medically at the time. I therefore asked myself the question: *What has to happen to stop this and reverse the problem from a medical point of view?* I also worked to recognize what the meaning of this could be, metaphysically.

Physically speaking, I knew that it was likely the fragile, newly grown blood vessels in the retina had ruptured and were leaking blood. So in order to control my focus and work with this, I began by getting into a relaxed state and communicating with my unconscious mind, telling it to: *Seal, heal, regress, and strengthen the blood vessels in the retina, providing a plentiful supply of oxygen and nutrients, as necessary.* I then kept visualizing this happening and repeating it as many times as I needed to, to avoid any negative or interrupting thought patterns... *Sealed, healed, healthy, and well.*

Next, I worked on getting to the root cause – the most important aspect. Metaphysically, our eyes reflect our ability to clearly see the past, present, and future. Eye problems, therefore, tend to reflect some distortion, fear, rage, or uncertainty about this.

For me personally, this has firmly resonated every time, particularly seeing red over a very distressing period of events. Being aware of it, and applying a specific resolution, seemed to assist me in the problem, dispersing it very quickly, as opposed to when I had applied nothing like this.

IMPORTANT - Please bear in mind that everyone is different, and there are many reasons why certain events happen, not necessarily diabetes related. So make sure that you have any symptoms or concerns checked and treated by your doctor and know precisely what you are dealing with, as well as the best course of action. Using positive mantras can dramatically help control your focus positively, and help manage and improve any symptoms or complications.

Some thoughts before we begin – Remember that any complications will be dramatically improved or even reversed by normal glucose control, so view this as a gradual process. That is why I have carefully laid the groundwork for this process throughout the preceding chapters in this book.

Use these positive thought patterns whenever you are symptomatic. It's best to use them when you are in a relaxed or trance-like state. Remember, when you are relaxed, or in a trance, the part of your mind that runs and maintains your body on auto pilot is most receptive.

Productive times to perform these mantras are when you are settling down, before you drift off to sleep, immediately on waking in the morning, and at other times throughout the day when you feel yourself daydreaming or drifting off. The patterns of proposed metaphysical emotional root causes and accompanying thought patterns will help you, no matter what time of day you apply them. They will also point you in the right direction by helping you find the necessary awareness to tackle the root problem.

Saying various mantras on a regular basis while doing the Body Scan meditation will significantly help. I have even recorded certain patterns with specific background music and played this at a low level when I'm drifting to sleep. Deep sleep is the time when our bodies are in their natural healing mode (as discussed in Chapter Six), so ensure that you are getting good-quality sleep to aid this process.

Be assured that no matter how and when you apply the mind-body connection, it is exceptionally powerful! Now is the time to really take on board that 'damaged nerve cells can sprout new growth'. Use the mind-body connection to encourage the body's infinite natural abilities.

Whether you visualize this, repeat it as a mantra to yourself, or both, whenever you do it and whatever details you say or visualize it doesn't matter – the fact that you are doing it and applying these methods in the most appropriate way for you is the key to helping overall health! Please remember that the root causes described are only a guide, and only you can ever really determine what the real, relevant emotional cause is for you personally. This guide is based on general metaphysical representations of our nervous system only. Have a look to see if the patterns described resonate with you in any way. Although nothing is 100 percent accurate, I personally find these patterns resonate (consciously) with at least 95 percent of clients I see in my practice.

If we keep delving further into root causes, we ultimately arrive at the negative emotion of *fear*. As discussed earlier, this is because every other negative emotion is derived from fear in some way. Aside from fear to protect us naturally, it is useless and dangerous to health. Remember that the body is a reflection or mirror of our inner thoughts and beliefs, because we are constantly sending messages and communicating with our body.

Ask yourself, *What possible thoughts may have resulted in this problem?* This will help create a higher self-awareness. Then instruct yourself to release these, do the work to let them go (using the resources in Chapter Five), and regularly repeat the suggested appropriate positive mantras.

It's important to mention that any current complaints you may have may be the consequence of an earlier complaint, or you may have had something for a long time and need to really think back to the emotional root cause of when that physical ailment began. To help clarify your awareness, keep asking yourself, *Why was that so, and why did it happen?* In this way, you will eventually get to the real root cause. Keep peeling back the layers of the onion until you reach the core!

I have intentionally left out the specific positive 'medical' mantras (apart from diabetes as a whole in Chapter Five and general complication avoidance in this chapter), because everyone is different with regards to what specifically needs to happen physically to assist in their individual treatment process.

To develop your own mantra, ask your physician specifically, 'What has to happen in order to successfully treat, restore, or fully reverse it?' If this question proves too challenging for your doctor, because they won't accept you can reverse it, you can ask 'How would "x" specifically function if nothing was deemed wrong with me?' Hopefully, your physician will wish to explain this, as their intention is to help you. If they are unable to appreciate your question, just ask them to at least humour you and explain that you want a positive focus.

Although these medical mantras are a useful support to assist in the healing/treatment process, the most important aspect is having an awareness of the emotional root cause and working on that, for all the reasons previously explained concerning the mind-body connection. This is what will always make the real difference!

With this list, I have done my best to represent the root cause of health conditions and mantras that can be applied, in general. If your specific condition or challenge does not appear in the list, read through and find the description that most closely approximates your unlisted complaint and use that as a guide. In this way, you can look at the wider meaning and put it into a specific context that resonates with you personally. Only you will know this, and deep down you will have the answers.

The subject of meta-physics is a branch of philosophy concerned with examining the relationship between mind and matter, and the first cause or principles of physical existence; the very core roots.

In relation to mind body medicine we are talking about the root cause of physical conditions; that which we cannot see, but rather feel and manifest.

In any case it is essential that we are aware of the very existence of metaphysical roots in order to successfully address, restore and fully explore them. We can then wholly appreciate and benefit from what our body is naturally capable of by way of our internal healing capacity.

As this table provides a strong guide as to the likely root causes of various conditions from the study of metaphysical connections and experiential research, it is most critical for you to establish a firm connection with your deep inner self. This involves developing a higher self-awareness and tapping further into your intuitive, more perceptive self. Certainly by working carefully through this book, expanding your philosophical thinking and adopting many of the resources and suggestions given, will help enhance this. Remember, you are the person to know your body best, and this comes with being able to trust your instinct and be honest with yourself.

NOTE: Some of the health challenges listed here have been adapted and extended from Louise Hay's original listings in her book *Heal Your Body*. Louise Hay is a well-known metaphysical lecturer, teacher, and best-selling author.

Challenge/ Organ	Potential root emotional problem/ bodily representation	Positive mantra/ awareness needed to assist, act upon, and release
Abscess/ boils/cuts/sores or inflammation	Fermenting thoughts over hurts and revenge. Suppressing anger and holding it in the body.	I allow my thoughts to be free. The past is over, and I am at peace. I can say if I am angry, and I know I can safely, outwardly express anger in a positive way, such as hitting the punch bag, exercising, singing about why I am angry in theatrical 'musical' and so on.
Aches	Longing for love, longing to be held.	I love and approve of myself. I am loving and lovable.
Allergies / food intolerances	Who or what are you allergic to? Denying your own power. What or who can't you stomach? Challenges with assimilating new ideas or experiences. Insecurity.	The world is safe and friendly. I am safe. I am at peace with life, everything happens for a reason, and I can take the positive lessons from all that occurs in my life.
Amenorrhea – absence of periods in reproductive age	Not wanting to be a woman. Dislike of the self, not feeling self-worth.	I am a great person, and I appreciate everything I am, flowing freely at all times. I am worthy of looking after myself at all times to restore harmony and perfect balance in my life.
Anorexia	Denying the self, extreme fear, self-hatred, and rejection.	It's safe to be me. I'm fantastic as I am. I choose to live. I choose joy and self-acceptance.
Anxiety	Not trusting the flow and process of life, some aspect of life you need to focus on and address to overcome.	I am safe. I love and approve of myself, and I trust the process of life. I have the resources to deal with everything I need and devote attention to.
Apathy – indifference – just not bothered.	Resistance to feeling. Deadening of the self, depressed mood – Deep-down fear.	It's safe to feel, and I open myself to life. I can happily embrace and experience life.

Challenge/ Organ	Potential root emotional problem/ bodily representation	Positive mantra/ awareness needed to assist, act upon, and release
Appetite – excessive (Although increased insulin can result in increased appetite, as well as being a potential hypo symptom – this refers to consistently wanting to noticeably overeat)	Fear, needing protection and comfort, masking or repressing true/deep emotions.	I am safe, and it is safe to feel. My feelings are normal and acceptable. I can change my feelings rather than binge.
Arteriosclerosis - thickening, hardening, and loss of elasticity of the arterial walls resulting in impaired blood circulation.	Resistance, tension. Hardened narrow-mindedness. Refusing to see good.	I am completely open to life and to joy. I choose to see with love and love life.
Atherosclerosis (Cholesterol) - A build-up of plaque (made from cholesterol, fatty, and cellular waste deposits, calcium, and fibrin) in the vessels. A form of Arteriosclerosis (hardening of the arteries).	Clogging the channels of joy, often through anger. Fear of accepting joy.	I choose to love life. My channels of joy are wide open, and it's safe to receive.
Blood pressure High	Long-standing emotional problem not solved – often masked by stress and anxiety.	I joyously release the past, I am at peace and have nothing to fear.
Blood pressure Low	Lack of love as a child. Defeatism. What's the use? It won't work, anyway. Tired of life.	I now choose to live a joyful life in the present. It's safe to do so, and I am in control to create positive and exciting change.
Bowel problems	Fear of letting go of the old. Fear of releasing that which we no longer need. Needing balance.	I freely release the old and openly welcome the new. I release any fear, as nothing holds me back. I have a perfect balance in life, whereby joy carries me forward into the new.
Bruises – ecchymoses	Little bumps in life. Self-punishment.	I love and cherish myself. I am kind and gentle to myself. All is well.

Challenge/ Organ	Potential root emotional problem/ bodily representation	Positive mantra/ awareness needed to assist, act upon, and release
Bulimia/dia-bulimia – (dia-bulimia is using diabetes as a tool to achieve the same effect as bulimia. It is just a label and a way of doing 'bulimia').	Hopeless terror or discontent. A frantic expression of self-hatred. Feelings of no other options – desperation and a missing need.	I am loved, nourished, and supported. I am safe, and I have choice. I am a great and resourceful person, capable of finding other ways, when I look. I have the ability to create positive change.
Candida – thrush/ yeast infections	Feeling very scattered and indecisive. Lots of frustration. Anger over making the wrong decisions. Denying your own needs and not supporting yourself.	I lovingly accept my decisions, knowing that I am free to change and everything happens for a reason to move us to where we're meant to be. I am safe. I choose to support, love, accept, and appreciate myself and others. I give myself permission to be all that I can be. I deserve the very best in life.
Circulation – Represents the ability to feel and express the emotions in positive ways	Repressing joyous, loving, happy feelings. Not feeling allowed/free or restricted to adequately express emotion in positive ways.	I am free to circulate joy, love, and happiness in all aspects of my life and universe. I love life, and I'm free to express it.
Colds (upper respiratory ailments)	Too much going on at once, mental confusion/ disorder. Small hurts, belief in getting 'x' number of colds/year.	I allow my mind to relax and be at peace. Clarity and harmony are within me and around me. All is well. I am fit, healthy, and well.
Coma	Fear. Escaping something or someone. Had enough – 'the only way to rest'.	We surround you with safety and love. We create a safe space for you to heal and live joyously. You are supported.
Cramps - (Although can be an indication of higher sugars and dehydration – focus on the reason for what is directly behind such a physical cause in the first place)	Tension, fear, holding on, gripping.	I relax and allow my mind to be peaceful. I can do all I need to do easily and effortlessly in good time.

Challenge/ Organ	Potential root emotional problem/ bodily representation	Positive mantra/ awareness needed to assist, act upon, and release
Depression	Anger and fear that you do not feel you have a right to have. Hopelessness.	I create my life. I can create positive change and release any fears and limitations. I can do whatever I focus my mind on.
Diabetes – Hyperglycaemia (high levels)	Longing for what might have been. A great need to control – perhaps something that has taken away your control – such as a form of loss. Deep sorrow. No sweetness left prior to diagnosis.	This moment is filled with joy, and I can enjoy everything I *do* have. I am always in control of my life and health. I choose to experience the sweetness of today and release the past.
Diabetes – Hypoglycaemia (low levels)	Overwhelmed – often by the burdens in life/events at the time. What's the use?	I am safe. I choose to make life light, easy, and joyful and give myself the break I deserve.
Dawn phenomenon – (High glucose on waking due to a natural glucose release during sleep as a result of certain hormones released so the body has the energy to wake).	This is a natural process that everyone experiences; however, enough insulin would ordinarily be released in order to store glucose in the cells. This therefore refers to needing to achieve more balance and harmony in all aspects of life. Needing safety and protection.	I am safe, I can rest easy. I have the resources and ability to find the balance and harmony I need to bring about peace and stability. I am safe, and I have the ultimate answers.
Diarrhoea	Fear. Rejection. Running off.	I am at peace with life and I create a perfectly balanced consumption, adjustment and removal of everything necessary in my life.
Edema/ retaining fluids, swelling	What or who won't you let go of?	I willingly let go of the past. It is safe for me to let go. I am free now.

Challenge/ Organ	Potential root emotional problem/ bodily representation	Positive mantra/ awareness needed to assist, act upon, and release
Eyes – Represent the capacity to see clearly	Often, something we don't want to see regarding the past, present, or future. Potentially seeing rage and fear. Pressure from long-standing hurts. Overwhelmed by it all.	I create a life with every-thing I love to look at, letting go of all rage and fear. I look forward to life and feel the joy, as I see clearly the past, present, and future. I am free of pressure, and it's perfectly safe for me to see. I see through loving eyes.
Fatigue (when inappropri-ate and unexplained)	Resistance, boredom, tired of life's challenges, lack of love for what one does.	I have my own life that I appreciate. It's for living with joy and enthusiasm. I can create and change this at any time, filling life with energy, fun, and enthusi-asm – where focus goes, energy flows. I choose to remove and unblock my energy channels, allowing them to flow freely.
Feet	Represent our understand-ing of ourselves, of life, of others – past, present, and future.	My understanding is clear, and I am willing to change with the times. I am safe.
Foot problems	Fear of the future and change. Not stepping forward in life. Resistance.	I move forward in life with joy and ease, embracing change, exploring all pos-sible routes. There's more than one way to move forward.
Flatulence (excess gas / gas pains). Also see aller-gies as a possibility.	Gripping. Fear. Undigested ideas.	I relax and let life flow through me with ease. I am safe, and trust in the process of life.
Gangrene	Mental morbidity. Drown-ing of joy with poisonous/ festering thoughts. Severe procrastination/mental stagnation.	I choose to take action, choosing harmonious thoughts, letting joy flow freely through me. I move to find positive change, Seek and I will find.
Gastritis	Prolonged uncertainty. A feeling of doom.	I love and approve of myself. I am safe.

Challenge/ Organ	Potential root emotional problem/ bodily representation	Positive mantra/ awareness needed to assist, act upon, and release
Genitals	Represents the masculine and feminine principles.	It is safe to be who I am. I love and appreciate all of my body. Nature is beautiful.
Genital problems	Worry about not being good enough. Irritated/ troubled by something or someone. Sexual guilt often regarding STI's.	I rejoice in my own expression of life. I am perfect just as I am. I love and approve of myself. I have the strength and ability to work through anything I need to. I can address the root and feel joy in all I do.
Heart	Represents the centre of love and security.	My heart beats joyously to the rhythm of love and life.
Heart Attack – myocardial infarction	Squeezing all the joy out of the heart in favour of money or position and so on.	I bring joy back into the centre of my heart, restoring balance and harmony back in my life. I express love throughout my life.
Heart problems (general)	Long-standing conflict and emotional problems. Lack of joy. Hardening of the heart. Belief in strain and stress.	I lovingly allow joy to easily and effortlessly flow through my mind and body experience. I have the courage, serenity, and ability to successfully work through and enjoy all that comes my way in life.
Heartburn	Clutching fear and anxiety.	I breathe freely and fully. I am safe, and I can rely on others. I trust and enjoy the process of life as I slow down (including speed of eating, and the pace of life).
Impotence	Sexual pressure, tension, guilt, social beliefs. Spite against a previous mate. Fear of the mother.	I allow the full power of my sexual principle to operate with ease and with joy. I choose to open fully the channels of joy. I am free to circulate love and joy in every part of my world.

Challenge/ Organ	Potential root emotional problem/ bodily representation	Positive mantra/ awareness needed to assist, act upon, and release
Incontinence	Emotional overflow. Years of controlling the emotions.	I am willing to feel. It is safe for me to express my emotions. I love and accept myself.
Incurable	Cannot be cured by outer means at this point. We must go deep within to stimulate the cure.	I have the power within to reverse this. Miracles happen every day, and I can embrace them and be one of them. I go deep within to dissolve the pattern that created this. I have the resources and the strength to do this.
Infection	Irritation, anger, annoy-ance.	I choose to be peace-ful and harmonious. I can easily let things go, because I have the power and strength to reject and better outer forces.
Viral Infection	Lack of joy flowing through life. Bitterness.	I lovingly allow joy to flow freely throughout my entire life. I love, appreci-ate, and accept myself. I am fully deserving of being free and happy.
Kidney Problems	Intensely troubled by criti-cism, disappointment, and failure. Shame. Reacting like a little kid.	Divine right universal action is always taking place in my life. Only good comes from each experi-ence. Everything happens for an ultimate positive reason, and I can take the learnings from this to successfully move on. It is safe to grow up. I am fulfilled.
Legs	Represent carrying us forward in life.	Life is for me, and it is for living. I have choices and options around me.
Lower leg problems	Fear of the future, not wanting to move.	I move forward with confidence, ease, and joy, knowing that all is well in my future. I can create and embrace what I want.

Challenge/ Organ	Potential root emotional problem/ bodily representation	Positive mantra/ awareness needed to assist, act upon, and release
Liver	Represents the seat of anger and core emotions.	Love, peace, and joy are what I know and focus on.
Liver problems	Feeling bad. Chronic complaining. Justifying fault-finding to deceive yourself.	I choose to live through the open space in my heart. I can confidently do everything I need to do to be fulfilled. I look for love and find it everywhere. I feel good about myself and all I choose to do.
Lung	The ability to take in life.	I take in life in perfect balance
Lung problems	Depression. Grief. Fear of taking in life. Not feeling worthy of living life fully.	I have the capacity to take in the fullness of life. I lovingly live life to the fullest.
Menstrual problems	Rejection of ones femininity. Guilt, fear. Belief that the genitals are dirty or sinful. Out of sync with life's balance.	I accept my full power as a woman and accept all my bodily processes are natural and normal. I love and approve of myself. I have created the perfect life balance I choose.
Constant negative suggestions from yourself or others. These represent some form of challenge to overcome.	There is something positive to learn here. There may be something you need to teach someone else and help others with, because you have the resources to do so. You may need challenges in order to think differently and fully protect yourself.	Everything happens for a reason. I choose to find the positive reason in this, as I have already rejected any negativity and successfully passed this challenge.
Nerves – Represent communication. They communicate the kind of messages you are circulating around your body. They are sensitive in detecting such messages (positive or negative).	Blockages or trouble in your internal communication.	I communicate easily and effortlessly, with warmth and joy. I know what I need to communicate for the best results.

Challenge/ Organ	Potential root emotional problem/ bodily representation	Positive mantra/ awareness needed to assist, act upon, and release
Numbness	Withholding love and consideration. Going dead mentally.	I share my feelings and love. I look towards doing what excites me. I'm receptive to the good that surrounds me, and I'm aware of all I need to be.
Overweight	Often represents stress and fear and the need for protection. Fear may be underlying anger and a resistance to forgive – the self or others.	I am always safe and secure, and I choose to take responsibility for my life, knowing that I create my own universe. I forgive myself and others. I now create my own life the way I want it, because I can.
Pancreas	Represents the sweetness of life	My life is sweet.
Pancreatitis	Rejection. Anger and frustration, because life seems to have lost its sweetness.	I love and approve of myself, and I alone create sweetness and joy in my life. It is there to be enjoyed, if I open to it.
Pre-menstrual syndrome (PMS)	Allowing confusion to reign. Giving power to outside influences. Rejection of the feminine processes.	I now choose to take charge of my mind and my life. I am a powerful, resourceful, and creative woman. I love who I am. All of my body functions in perfect harmony.
Seizures	Running away from the family – yours or another, the self, from life.	I am at home in the universe. I am safe, secure, and understood.
Skin	Protects our individuality – a sense organ.	I feel safe to be me. I am confident in my own skin and happy with who I am.
Skin – boils, sores, inflammation, 'itis'	Indications of anger expressing in the body due to being supressed – a fear of anger.	I can safely express and release any anger in my body easily and effortlessly. It is safe for me to feel emotion and let it out – it serves no purpose. I express love and joy, as I see only 'positive' self-intentions for the behaviours around me.

Challenge/ Organ	Potential root emotional problem/ bodily representation	Positive mantra/ awareness needed to assist, act upon, and release
Stomach	Holds nourishment, digests ideas.	I digest life with ease.
Stomach problems – generic	Dread, fear, inability to adjust or conform to the new.	Life agrees with me. I can easily adjust to the new and embrace all that is ahead. All is well.
Stroke – cerebrovascular accident (CVA)	Resistance. Strong reluctance to change – potential rejection of life. Lacking joy flowing freely.	Life is change, I am flexible and dynamic to embrace and enjoy the new. I accept life – past, present, and future.
Mini stroke – Transient Ischemic Attack (TIA)	Periodic restriction and reluctance to openly feel joy, growing resistance. A need for inner change and contentment.	I freely express and receive joy. I awaken new life within me, and I flow freely. Joyous new ideas are floating freely within me, and I now choose to embrace them.
Thyroid	Potential feelings of humiliation in terms of never getting to do what one really wants.	I let go of old limitations and move towards the new, expressing myself freely and creatively.
Hyperthyroidism	Rage/ hurt at being left out.	I am at the centre of life. I approve of myself and all that I see.
Hypothyroidism	Feeling hopelessly stifled/ stuck, giving up.	I create a new life with new rules that wholly support me.
Teeth – Represent decisions Teeth problems	Long standing indecisive-ness. Challenges over decisions, unfortunate decision. Too analytical to actually commit to a decision.	I make my decisions based on the truth. I can trust and wholeheartedly believe in the decisions I make. I make this decision with conviction.
Tongue	Represents the ability to taste the pleasures of life with joy and ease.	I enjoy all of my life and all it gives me, as I know everything is for a reason to ultimately and posi-tively support me.

Challenge/ Organ	Potential root emotional problem/ bodily representation	Positive mantra/ awareness needed to assist, act upon, and release
Urinary infections (upper and lower UTI's)	Anxiety. Holding onto ideas. Fear of letting go. Pissed off, irritated by people or things, but most often at the opposite sex or sexual partner.	I let go of any irritations and limitations. I have more to enjoy and focus on. I am willing to change. I love and approve of myself. I easily and effort-lessly release the old and welcome the new in my life. I am safe, and it is safe let go.

In addition to the above, I have composed a generic medical mantra to assist in improving and avoiding diabetes complications. You can use this as often as you like. It is also useful to use with the Body Scan meditation:

I have plenty of free-flowing oxygen and nutrients circulating easily and effortlessly throughout my entire body, travelling through strong healthy blood vessels, supporting clear and flexible arteries.

I have perfect internal stability and balance, in which my immune system thrives, providing strength, resilience, and health. I have the optimal balance of hormones, fluids, acids, and enzymes to regulate natural, full health and well-being.

My blood supply is healthy and free flowing to every organ, ensuring optimum function, health, and healing, as I am strong, healthy, energetic, and well, supporting my ability to live freely.

I hope this chapter assists you in finding the positive inspiration you need to address any potential complications of diabetes. Contrary to popular belief – medical or mass media – diabetes never needs to be about doom and gloom. There's plenty you can do to prevent complications, stop them, and dare I say it, reverse them. You know the score by now – it's all a mind-set!

CHAPTER EIGHT SUMMARY

- Although complications can be distressing, we can do plenty!
- Following any diagnosis, making *gradual* improvements is crucial.
- Although we know how we need to ultimately think and act to get the results we want, it's key to express emotions first (safely).

- Releasing natural negative energy and emotion first will pave the way for positively retuning your focus and the best outcome.
- A positive focus and coping method is key.
- Specific positive 'mantras' can be applied to proactively redirect our focus for a positive physical outcome.
- These positive thought patterns can help you to trace and establish likely emotional root causes behind specific complications.
- You can apply medical mantras to enhance physical healing.
- Ask your doctor to explain what needs to happen physically to reverse your challenge.
- You can use the medical mantra given to avoid and assist in generally healing complications - use in meditation and trance.
- There's plenty you can do to prevent, stop, and reverse complications. Never give up, because you're better than that.

Piecing It All Together and Getting Exactly What You Want

Deep down, most of us have an idea of what we want in life, but it can be all too easy to lose sight of this, becoming unfocused, unmotivated, or just distracted by life itself. The key to avoiding all this is to know exactly what we want by having a precise outcome.

If you think about it, the people who know exactly what they want from the very outset and commit to that decision always seem to get exactly what they want sooner or later, in one way or another. Often, you can usually spot this in people, because they have a strong determination and everything focused on it.

If I've ever *really* wanted something in life, I've got it – not in a privileged or self-entitled way, but because without any question I knew my outcome and set my mind on it. The times that I have found myself distracted, not wholly congruent about something, or slightly off course in life, I haven't got what I want.

What's interesting about this is that if I've ever *thought* I wanted something but didn't deep down want it, or believed I wasn't really worthy of it, I've never got it! This tells us a lot about where our real drive and focus comes from and how knowing that makes all the difference in the results we get in life. Quite simply we have to wholeheartedly, deep down want something for it to give us enough determination and motivation to go out there and get it.

As I have shown throughout this book, there are a variety of neurological techniques we can apply to ensure we get exactly what we want. I will discuss how in this chapter.

First of all, we've pretty much established that for anything to be successful we need a strong, prioritized motivation behind it. It has to be important enough to us, or we simply won't be focused or motivated enough to take action and do anything about it.

In some cases, we may need to be seriously disturbed about something before we act. A common example is when people have to experience a serious health threat or heart attack in order to make them take action to lose weight. Alternatively, we might be already naturally focused on our intention, such as losing weight to be healthy, look trimmer for a wedding outfit or photo shoot, or run a marathon.

Bottom line: We need to be bothered enough by something and have a compelling reason to act and remain positively motivated in order to reach our goal.

In my own life, for instance, if I had a goal to get super physically fit at the moment, it would be a total waste of time, because although that would be nice, it's just not important enough to me right now. I would have no compelling reason, because my BMI and general health is good and I'm perfectly happy as I am, deep down. However, if I suddenly decided to take part in the notorious Iron Man triathlon, I might suddenly develop a motivation to get in peak physical fitness and tone up, because of having a greater purpose and incentive to do so!

One way to find out how motivated we are about something is to ask ourselves the following question and write down the answers very quickly in list form:

'What's most important to you about living?'

1. ....

2. ....

3. ....

4. ....

5. ....

6. ....

7. ....

8. ....

Keep listing any more that come to you, until you begin repeating the same ones.

Generally speaking the first things that come to mind (the top of your list) are most likely to reflect your inner order of importance, and that's what we're really interested in.

So on that note, did health or your representation of health come anywhere near or at the top of your list? Is health important enough to you at the moment to keep you motivated and doing something about it?

In terms of your list, the higher you place health, or your representation of health, on the list, the better, as this signifies how important health generally is to you! The more important it is, the more motivation you will have to achieve your health goals. This is because it is in your values – the things that are important to you, and ultimately provide your motivation to take action.

If it's a little lower down than you'd have hoped, and you'd like a bit more motivation, have a think about your higher intention and motivation behind doing what you want to do. Also read on through the rest of this chapter, as it will help you get to what you specifically want.

If you still have challenges with your motivation and values, a good clinical hypnotherapist or NLP Master Practitioner or Coach should be able to assist you in this, if you explain that you would like to change your values regarding your health in order to increase your motivation (refer to the Resources section for guidance on the best places to find certified hypnotherapists and NLP practitioners).

If you placed health high on your list already, you'll likely experience exceptional results if you apply all the resources throughout this book and the information in this chapter. Keep focused, and go for it! As with everything, there are certain steps that can help to make a goal or idea a reality. If we carefully apply all these steps, there's every reason we can get exactly what we want, irrespective of any challenges and general life hurdles along the way.

I've definitely had plenty of challenges and bumps along the road that I've had to overcome in order to successfully get my outcome. Some are even hard to imagine now, and that's not something I say lightly. So prepare yourself to start getting the things you want from life. Just make sure you really believe you deserve them. If not, it's a limitation with a deeper emotional root behind it (see Chapter Five).

Keys to Achieving Your Goal

When you've gone through all these steps, keep them in mind every day and regularly ask yourself upon waking:

What has to happen today in order for me to achieve my goal or make sure that I take even more steps closer to achieving it?

1. **Make it very specific.**
    Have a precise knowledge of what your goal is and how you're going to achieve it. For example, just saying 'I'm going to improve my sugar levels' isn't specific enough. What range are you aiming for? How are you going to do this? And for what purpose are you going to do this? What's your motivation?

2. **Make it measurable.**
    How will you know when you have successfully achieved your goal? What has to happen for you to know that you have achieved this? What evidence do you need? How can you measure your success, what can you judge it on? For example, do you need to have had a consistent HbA1c of a certain number, such as 6 percent, with great energy levels, a certain medication dosage, and overall great health for a period of time? What is the specific benchmark that means you have got what you want?

3. **Imagine your goal as if it has come true right now.**
    Get a feel for this and program it into your mind, so you really know your outcome. Use all your senses to do this.
    - See what you can see when you have already achieved your goal.
    - Hear what you can hear. Are you saying anything to yourself, such as, *Yes! I've done it!* or is someone else congratulating you, or complimenting you on this? This might even be your doctor or a loved one?
    - Now feel the emotions that you feel when you have achieved your goal. Are you happy, laughing, excited, overwhelmed, amazed, and so on?
    - Are there any specific scents present? Are you in a specific place – perhaps the doctor's surgery or at your home?

- Are there any specific tastes present? Are you having a drink or something to eat as a celebration?

This is specific to you. It is about how your mind chooses to present this to you. However, make sure you use all your senses and make this as specific as possible, with as much detail and clarity as you can. You know how visualization works! (Chapter Five)

4. **Make sure you have reasonable and realistic steps with plenty of alternatives to achieve this, should you need them.**
   - Do you have the right resources and support you need to achieve your goal?
   - Have you allowed for a sensible period of time to achieve this?
   - Do you have the right motivation and mind-set needed?
   - Is your focus and belief wholeheartedly there?
   - Have you got other options and ways to achieve your goal?
   - What other information and resources can you access?
   - What other support can you get, should any challenges arise?

5. **Allow time, and be specific.**
   All too often, we say we want to achieve something, but we either don't allow the necessary time to do this, or it goes on and on, meaning that we never really commit to an outcome. For example, if I didn't have a precise outcome, I may be writing this book for the rest of my life!

   On that note: Be realistic but also specific. Ask your unconscious mind very quickly exactly when you will achieve this – which month, date, and year? This way you will certainly know your outcome and your mind knows exactly where to focus.

   Never be afraid to commit to a date. Trust yourself. You will always release diabetes emotionally first, which is something you will feel, *then* follows the physical retraining of your body to function independently and the constant progression back to full health. So just keep this in mind when your specific date comes round!

   If you apply all of the aforementioned steps thoroughly, you'll embed them into your neurology, so that you become focused – and, as you know by now, where focus and attention go, energy and results certainly follow, which is exactly what you want!

Remember also how our minds work, and visualize your goal with clarity and detail. The part of our mind that runs and maintains our body is unable to distinguish between what is 'real' and what is 'not real'. Therefore, knowing our outcome can quite literally be positively programmed and pre-set into our entire neurology to achieve the precise results we want.

We can also take our goals one step further, in order to embed these into our future. Although we tend to think of a 'memory' as 'a past memory', we can also have 'future memories', or 'strong visions' if you like. A memory is just the process in which we encode, store, and retrieve information that is outside our present world, so in this respect we can create a very specific 'future memory'.

How to Pre-Determine and Establish Your Goal as a Future Memory

Go back to Step 3 above, imagine your goal 'as if' it has already happened. Imagine the last step that has to happen in order for you to know you have successfully achieved this goal. How do you know it has come true?

- See clearly what you can see with as much detail as possible – Who or what is there? Where are you? What are you wearing? What else can you see around you?
- Hear what you can hear – Are there any apparent noises? Is anyone saying anything to you? Are you saying something to yourself?
- How do you feel? – Is this an internal feeling, or are you displaying your emotions physically or externally in some way?
- What scents do you smell?
- What tastes do you taste?
  Use all your available senses to make this experience as prominent, real, detailed, and clear as possible.

Now step out of this experience.

Imagine you are looking at this experience as if it is a photograph you are holding in your hand. As you look at this photograph, see it with excitement and joy as something that has already happened. Keep focused on those associated feelings, and take three long, deep breaths (in through your nose and out through your mouth), and feel a positive surge of energy rush through you, down your arms, and into the photo you are holding of this future memory. Keep hold of this positively charged photograph.

Prepare to travel into your future.

Now clutching this energized photograph, close your eyes and imagine drifting in a hot air balloon basket (like in the Chapter Five 'Emotional Release' techniques). Start rising in the balloon, and head out towards your future. Travel out into the future until you feel you have reached the specific point at which you will have reached your goal (the date you came up with in Step 5 above).

Stop, and hover above this specific time.

Now gently drop your photographed future memory down into this part of your future life. See it float down, and slot in perfectly! As you do this, just hear it CLICK into place, as it now becomes locked into your future. As you do this, hear the sound of a lock or a door closed tight.

Travel back to the present.

Once you've done this, as you travel back to the present in your balloon, notice how when you glance down, everything else in your life adjusts accordingly, in order to support you in having successfully already achieved this future memory. You notice all other events align to support your goal becoming a reality.

Drift back into your body and enjoy.

Once you are back to the present, lower your balloon, get out, and drift back into your body. Open your eyes, and enjoy the feeling that you have affirmed a future memory, whereby you will now take all the necessary steps to get to this and embrace it.

NOTE: If you have any challenges following this process, you could ask someone close to assist you by reading it out, or you can experience an audio version of the visualization by visiting www.dr-em.co.uk under Making Your Goal A Real Outcome.

This goal is now heavily imprinted in your entire neurology through every one of your senses, and once again, you know how the mind-body connection works, so there's a lot to be excited about! I've done this type of work with many people, myself included, and I've always known it to work when done properly. Although some people might find this technique a little 'out there', this really depends on how much you can appreciate the science and workings of our neurology. Anyone who wants to, can and will experience phenomenal results, but it all starts with the right mind-set.

The General Keys to Success

Below are some of the general keys to success that can be applied to anything! These will always help massively when applied throughout life, and even when you already know them, they are still great to be reminded of and reinforced.

Know your outcome specifically.

I'm guessing you've just done that one!

Take action.

Although this sounds an obvious one, it's still easy to dismiss. I think that at times we've all been guilty of it, too. We might have a great opportunity or plan, but we don't always take the action necessary to really make it happen. Classic examples of this are in business, when people set up great websites with excellent business potential that look fantastic, then sit back and expect visitors and hits to automatically come. Unless we take necessary action in doing the hard work of promoting and marketing it, it never happens!

Have behavioural and mental flexibility.

Behavioural and mental flexibility are vital to success. To my mind, with all-round flexibility anything is possible, as being flexible helps put you in control of the situation. I've always got (eventually) what I've wanted by being flexible and thinking outside the box.

It's about never taking no for an answer, because there's usually another way to get over obstacles. There's always more than one way of doing something, no matter how unconventional it may seem – we just have to think about it. If it's not a problem for you, it doesn't have to be a problem for others, then we're all happy.

Life throws up plenty of challenges and natural obstacles from time to time, but if we have flexible thinking and behaviour, we can more often than not easily solve our challenges.

A key in how to do this is by using 'lateral/ logical thinking'. Start by ask yourself the question:

What is the main purpose, point, and intention of something in the first place? What's the bigger picture?

Once you get to this, ask yourself:

What are other examples of this – other ways/alternatives in which I could achieve the same thing?

Think about challenges in the past, and how if you or someone else had flexible thinking and behaviour at the time what a different and more productive outcome you could have potentially got. It's just about thinking differently and other ways of looking at something. What factors can you change to make something seem better or more suitable? What else can you do about it?

You may have heard the following story, but it's a great one where flexibility is concerned.

It all started by someone throwing some bread in the park for the birds. As you can imagine, there were too many birds for the amount of bread. Whilst all the other birds were trying to get as many pieces as they could, there was one bird who just took one piece and waited for the other birds to finish and leave. This particular bird then got the one saved piece and dropped it into the lake and watched closely. The bird had waited for a fish to come to the surface and then got the fish. The bird also managed to get this one piece of bread back and repeated the process. So through some great flexibility, this bird suddenly created a feast from a tiny amount of food.

The more flexibility any of us display in our thinking, creativity, and behaviour, the more options and solutions we will create for ourselves to get a better outcome. Imagine if the patients in Chapter Seven case studies were so inflexible in their thinking and behaviour that they were unable to conceive of any other treatment options – options that incidentally saved their lives.

Have great observation and awareness skills.

Being aware and noticing things helps you stay several steps ahead and makes it much easier to figure out when something might be wrong. You can then work out exactly what you need to change to bring about better results. You can do this by trusting and listening carefully to your deep inner voice – your gut feeling and intuition. Learning to meditate, applying peripheral vision to remain calm but focused (explained in Chapter Five), and finding other ways to give yourself head space will also increase your awareness skills, allowing you to sense things before they happen through greater observation skills.

It's useful to practise seeing things from another person's point of view by taking time to step into their shoes. In this way, you become really good at seeing things from other perspectives. This helps you pick up on much more around you, about yourself, or about other people, so you can avoid situations that may not be beneficial to you.

Maintain a great physiology and psychology of excellence.

It's important to be mindful of how we look, in terms of our posture, facial expressions, and body language. For example, avoid slumping, continually yawning, or frowning; instead, smile, stand, or sit up straight, and look alert, because how we hold ourselves also affects how we feel. You don't tend to see happy or excited people who slump and look down in the mouth with a continuous frown. Holding a 'physiology of excellence' is a must for encouraging good health.

A Physiology of Excellence

A recent example of the effects of physiology on well-being occurred when we delivered a 'Well-Being in the Workplace' professional teacher training in health and well-being in the UK. In fact, I think we are both still feeling stunned by it...

On our arrival, we were greeted (if you can call it that) by one of the primary school teachers. She plodded towards us, dragging her feet, no smile, head towards the floor, and shoulders slumped (and this wasn't down to any disability, as I'd checked beforehand). When we introduced ourselves and asked if she'd had a good day, in a very flat voice she answered, 'Better now that's over.'

This was before we had even met the rest of the group, who much to our disbelief, carried the same general physiology and attitude. What's really interesting here is that these people also projected profuse negativity about everything we had to say (which was very positive and proactive).

Fortunately, a small minority of the group, including the head teacher, had an upbeat physiology. They sat up straight yet relaxed, smiled, looked alert, and had a positive attitude. Interestingly it was these people who got a lot out of the training and continually get great results in their professional and personal lives, despite having their challenges too!

So physiology is really important in terms of expressing how we feel, what we project to the world, and the results we get. You only have to think of all the successful, happy people you know. Do you ever see them looking or behaving in the same way as most of the teachers I've described? Incidentally, after explaining the mind body connection, and using my results as one of many examples, one teacher directly said to me (rudely with offence intended) "I don't believe you can stop diabetes. My reply... 'Exactly, and *you* wouldn't!... I'm guessing you get exactly where that was going!

Having a 'psychology of excellence' simply means remaining in control of our thoughts and emotions in order to control and maintain our internal and external state (our mood).

This is important because although we know all too well that not everything in life is cheerful, and tragic things can happen, we still need to keep an overall positive outlook so we can nevertheless be resourceful and get the best outcome possible.

Utilizing an Excellent Physiology and Psychology

I know first-hand how these two factors of maintaining an excellent physiology and psychology makes all the difference. I remember one occasion, our first training with a new business. The room was full of executives, and the managing director, human resources, and operations manager sat at the back of the room, judging everything.

I wasn't feeling my best. I'd not slept the night before, was feeling extremely nauseous, and to top it off had come down with a rare cold, and a bad one at that. So all I wanted to do was curl up in the hotel room and go to sleep! However, it was 5am, and we had to be up preparing for an early start and late finish. At the same time, I also knew we needed to make an excellent impression and get certain results from this training, because a lot of future business and our reputation depended on it.

I needed to pull everything out of the bag, including all of the steps for success I've described earlier, particularly the last ones, which successfully got me through the day so that I could actually enjoy it, too. In changing my focus and state to everything I wanted it to be, I positively distracted my mind, creating positive chemical and physical changes. That resulted in me enjoying the day, and everything being a great success. So again all the above steps are well worth applying for great results all round!

This chapter helps us to get specific and reinforce what we really want, how to get it, and how to account for all else successfully along the way. It may also help you discover if you *really* don't want something enough, too. So whatever you do want from life, go out and get it, because nothing has to stop you – especially diabetes!

CHAPTER NINE SUMMARY

- It can be easy to lose sight of the things we really want in life. To avoid this we need to have a precise outcome.
- If we ever *think* we want something but don't deep down, we'll never get it, because we will lack the drive and motivation necessary. Having deep-down drive makes all the difference to the results we can get. We *have* to be bothered enough!
- You can check on your motivation levels by working out your values. Your values are what is important to you and, of course, this is what gives you the motivation to act.
- The more something is consciously and unconsciously important to you in the relevant context (life, work, relationships, and so on), the more motivation and drive you will have to achieve your goal.
- Strong visualization aids programming your goal into your entire neurology, so that your conscious and unconscious mind know where to focus. You can create a future memory of your goal to ensure the path of it becoming a reality.
- The principle keys to success make an enormous difference in the results we can get.
- Whatever you want from life, you can go out and get it; diabetes is no barrier!

A Final Word

By applying and road testing everything in this book personally and professionally, I have experienced and witnessed some amazing results when it comes to diabetes. My aim has been to provide you with all the resources and support to do exactly the same.

Above all else I sincerely hope to assist in positively changing the perception and experience of diabetes, from the dis-ease the rest of the world currently knows into something radically different: a problem of the past!

What one person can do, so can another ... if they allow the possibility.

Inevitably, you will encounter sceptics and people unable to comprehend mind-body medicine – that includes people you know and deem intelligent, who may not share your excitement (you've read Chapter Seven!). If that's the case, maintain an indestructible, strong, and determined mind-set in order to ensure your continued success. Remember: Every successful person encounters doubters; it's just part of the process and generally indicates that you're doing something right.

Speaking of doubters or 'negitudes', I did finally find the answer to what I was so desperately seeking back in my late teens. It was never easy riding the storm, but my tiresome journey of harrowing symptoms did come to an end. By having the guts and tenacity to keep pushing on, trusting myself that I knew my body best, that *this was about more than just diabetes*, I got the right team, the people who were going to help and support me in my quest. This fantastic team, assisted me in looking way beyond the surface to get the necessary results.

The process wasn't easy or particularly comfortable, but I confronted these challenges using every personal resource I had available, because I knew we were close. Then finally, I was enlightened. I have Wilson's dis-ease: a rare genetic condition, whereby copper had been accumulating in my body since birth so that by my late teens it was effectively poisoning me. At this stage, Wilson's dis-ease begins to affect the liver and brain, not to mention play havoc with diabetes.

Suddenly, everything began to fall into place – why what happened to me happened. I may well not have even written this book otherwise. My life took a different direction because it had to, but that was the key. Talk about everything happening for a higher purpose, irrespective of it being good or not at the time!

Although it took some time, patience, and dedication to get things right, and I had to work hard to bring both conditions back under control, things were all about to change in a very positive way.

My health changed beyond recognition, going from strength to strength, because I was aware of what I was *really* dealing with. Even though Wilson's dis-ease is regarded as another life-long condition, as far as I'm concerned, it's just another progressive re-correction. Too much copper (a metal) in-side me that I can't excrete naturally, accumulating from birth – interesting, metaphysically. And that, of course, is the key to unlock all else.

In actual fact, this was just the beginning of my journey – only this time, the engine was firing on all cylinders; there was nothing to hold me back, other than myself. I could do what was important to me, take charge of the controls, step on the accelerator, and enjoy the ride.

IN CONCLUSION: Based on what human neurology is infinitely capable of, everything is a possibility. It's all out there, waiting to be discovered: the means to keep moving forward and making progress. Those who fail to grasp this fact are only choosing to engage in self-limitation, and can't 'impossible' actually read 'I'm possible', anyway? Perhaps, only if we want it to. On that note, life is for exploring and discovering the new. Where would we be today if it wasn't? That's the only scary thing here. Wishing you the absolute best in your own personal journey. Go for it, and enjoy the process always in the knowledge of your ultimate outcome. What's the worst that can happen? Or should I say, what's the best thing that can happen? That's right!

CHAPTER TEN SUMMARY

- Wholeheartedly believe in yourself, have a solid and specific plan, apply the tips and resources throughout this book, and seriously go for it, knowing your outcome all the way!
- Now you're at the controls, you can choose to accelerate and fly.
- Now you can draw your own conclusion. Whatever you choose to seek, need to learn, and wherever you choose to find value – it's all in there, so get the best for you.

Troubleshooting Guide
Help With Getting to the Root of Unexplained Conundrums When Things Go Astray

From time to time, we all have little bumps along the way, and although there's always a deep-seated root behind it that needs resolving, this root may be causing another physical reaction that might be causing something with diabetes to go astray.

For example, there have been several times when, despite the fact I've been eating well and injecting accordingly, my blood sugar levels have been elevated, seemingly for no apparent reason. As it turned out, I was extremely tired and overworked, which resulted in my adrenaline production going into overdrive to keep me going. As adrenaline causes blood sugar levels to rise, you can see what was happening, despite all that I was doing to keep on top of things.

This was the physical cause, but on a larger scale, I realized that the real root cause was that my life was out of balance in terms of the workload and type of work I was doing. So although we might not immediately be aware of the real root cause, it can nevertheless result in other physical reactions that then cause something to go off kilter with diabetes.

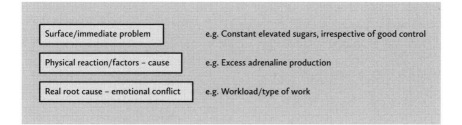

This troubleshooting guide offers help by prompting you to think about other factors, such as physical reactions that could be taking place or making things go awry. This may help uncover the real root cause underlying the 'physical' problem.

Checklist of Possibilities For Things Going Astray

Are you eating enough?

For our bodies to function properly, they need enough calories to give us energy. So never be afraid to eat – just eat more of the right things. This is especially the case if you experience 'dawn phenomenon'. Although your blood sugar may be elevated in the morning, the body still needs some food to balance this. Just have a bit of something with lower sugar, such as eggs, light toast, or low-carbohydrate granola, to give things a kick-start.

Is your body trying to protect your energy levels and keep you alert for any reason by stimulating production of more adrenaline?

Adrenaline naturally elevates sugar levels, and even more so when your body requires more adrenaline in order to keep you awake and alert. It signals that we need to relax and get some good rest to calm this down, especially after sleep deprivation.

There have been times when I (or Johnny, my partner) have been required to work in different countries, and although my sugars have been in a good range, when Johnny has been away and I've been by myself for some time, my sugars are naturally always more elevated (all things being equal, otherwise). This is simply because of having more adrenaline to keep more alert than usual, and more things to get done in our practice.

In addition to this, when I train and lecture for lengthy periods, it can be pretty intense in terms of performance and energy levels, so again my sugars are slightly more elevated than usual. Although they are still in a normal range because I know how to control this, it could be easy to let them become elevated outside that normal range, without knowing what I needed to do, so it's always worth bearing in mind similar factors.

Have your activity levels declined or increased without realizing it?

If you've had a pretty physically demanding job or project you've been working on (even renovating a house, or a period of extra-long shifts, or the like) and then either changed jobs, resumed regular hours, or completed your project, you may have suddenly ended up using far less energy without even realizing it (or the reverse). This could then naturally be having an impact on sugar levels as the body becomes accustomed to responding to a certain routine. It might just be a case of finding a replacement for whatever might have changed, or working out any other life changes that might need balancing.

Could you be secretly overeating without realizing it?

By this I don't mean eating behind closed doors and hiding it from people; I'm referring to eating extra food without realizing it. For example, is anyone giving you extra portions of food (particularly parents or loved ones who enjoy feeding you up)? Do you serve large portions yourself or eat the kids' leftovers before your own meal? Are you picking and snacking more than you realize? Sugar, carbs, and calories add up here and there. Do you find you have less time to sit and eat proper meals? Have you been grabbing and eating on the go?

This can often mean a lot of extra processed foods with hidden ingredients that can impact sugar levels. Even if you do manage to grab healthy food, this can also increase stress levels in terms of feeling more rushed, resulting in the body secreting increased adrenaline, and in turn, indirectly causing increased blood sugar levels.

Do you have enough insulin in your system?

Depending on your personal regime and insulin choices, your existing insulin could have run out. Are you familiar with your 'active insulin time'? This is roughly how long it is effective within your body? You may need to increase your injection frequency or insulin type. Also, has your insulin been going in properly? I know all too well how the injection pen can (for various reasons) become blocked and not administer the units you think it has. Pumps aren't infallible, either, so it's worth checking everything is working properly.

Is your particular medication suiting you?

Some medications have a better effect than others, so it might be worth exploring all other options and regimes to suit you best.

Have you been travelling or not slept?

When it comes to blood sugar levels, I've found travelling or getting less sleep can result in either higher or lower sugars. It's worth keeping in mind the importance of good sleep and catching up on this wherever possible.

When you travel, also bear in mind that you may be crossing different time zones. This can sometimes mean that you need to increase or decrease insulin a little, and administer in smaller more regular doses, until you settle into the new time zone.

Another consideration is the different foods you eat when you travel, from food on the plane to motorway services, not to mention in the particular country you might be visiting. For example, if you travel to the United States or United Arab Emirates, you will find some amazing dishes on the menus. But even when you are careful and conscientious about what you eat, certain products appear to be naturally sweeter than in the UK or Europe, even basics like bread, sauces, milk, cheeses, and cereals/porridge. In some hot climates, the range of vegetables can be different, too. If that's the case, do your best to get your nutrients where you can, and be mindful of the differences in what appear to be similar products.

Unfortunately, no matter where you are in the world, when it comes to eating out, good-quality food and food for special diets tend to cost more. Creativity and resourcefulness are often useful here.

Could you have any background infection your body is fighting?

As you already know, if you are fighting an infection this can easily knock your diabetes off kilter? When this has happened to me in the past, once I've sorted out any other problem, my sugars have always returned to normal pretty quickly. The types of infections I am referring to include UTIs, colds, shingles, tooth abscesses, and in my case, Wilson's disease. Always be careful that diabetes doesn't mask something unrelated.

Could you have a hormone imbalance that needs addressing? Are you taking other medication, contraceptives, herbal pills, stimulants (including excess coffee) that could be having a detrimental impact?

Are there any stressful events coming up?

If you have upcoming stressful events, you may have put these in the back of your mind consciously, but your unconscious (which controls your body physically) has not forgotten and will manifest the stress in one way or another. Alternatively, it could be that you are sensing something on the horizon that may be negative or causing you anxiety.

Speaking for myself, I have a pretty acute awareness and tend to detect things before they happen, because I sense them. This often manifests physically as an internal niggle and slightly elevated sugars for no apparent reason – well, until a week or so before. Remember how our minds work. We don't have to be directly thinking about something for it to affect us physically!

Be aware that certain things may be distracting you, so be mindful of your natural stress response, work out how you can best manage it, and adjust things accordingly.

Are you drinking enough fluids? – No, I don't mean alcohol!

We need good hydration in order for our cells and organs to function properly, so drink plenty of water. Dehydration never helps stabilize diabetes!

Are you drinking certain drinks that may be causing an unwanted side-effect?

Beverages like energy drinks often contain caffeine, a stimulant that can impact increasing blood sugar levels without you realizing it – even when they are marked 'sugar free'. These energy drinks can also add to kidney damage! 'No *added* sugar' drinks can also contain quite a lot of sugar, even though it might be natural sugar, it still counts.

Have you been consuming a lot of 'sugar free' or 'diet foods'?

A lot of 'sugar free', 'Diet', or 'No Added Sugar' foods contain 'sugar alcohols', which are often not taken into account when counting sugars, because they are hard for the body to digest and therefore effect blood sugars *less* than other carbohydrates. However, note: They can still elevate sugar levels, despite the purpose of 'sugar free' foods. Therefore remember to *subtract half* the amount in grams of sugar alcohols listed,[24] from the total amount of carbohydrates. This is why it's best to eat more foods that are naturally lower in carbohydrates, in order to keep a good balance and avoid too much artificial sweetener. The latter can also have a laxative affect, which can in turn negatively affect blood sugars.

Have your insulin or meds been in the sun, or could they be out of date?

Heat and expired dates can render your medications ineffective, and you may not realize you have a problem until they stop working. For example, during trips to hot locations in Nevada in the United States, and more recently in the United Arab Emirates, I had to throw away numerous insulin pens because the insulin had started to bubble and evaporate out of the pen. In addition, my BM machine was often too overheated to switch on! I did use a cooler bag, but this soon heated up, too! Talk about 'British' insulin – clearly, it was not familiar with the sun! Seriously, though, pay attention to this, even if you have to ask for an ice bucket to put insulin in at the beach. It helps.

Are you injecting enough insulin or medication for the current circumstances?

Although I now require very low doses of insulin, I still have to increase the amounts I inject during times of stress, bereavement, or for whatever reason it becomes necessary. Sometimes, you have to accept that you might need to temporarily adjust things and take your foot off the peddle a little until you are ready to get back on track. It's normal. Always listen to your body. Everything happens for a reason, so always trust yourself, and give yourself a break if you need to!

I hope the above troubleshooting suggestions help. I've experienced most of the situations described here at some point, but these prompts are really there to see if anything rings a bell so you can make an adjustment, or help uncover any other emotional roots that were not apparent or immediately obvious. I want to reiterate: It's important to always consult your specialist, so that you can talk through and work out any specifics or any potential issues that I haven't mentioned here.

Resources

PLEASE NOTE: This section is designed to offer some useful resources for you to draw on and will give you a sense of where to start looking. It does not necessarily contain all my own personal recommendations – I always recommend that you do your own research and find what works best for you.

From personal knowledge and experience, I can say that accreditations and qualifications do not always denote excellence in a practitioner; instead, seek testimonials from others whom you trust and speak to the practitioner first, if possible. This way you'll soon gauge if they are right for you or not.

ABNLP – American Board of Hypnotherapy and Neuro Linguistic Programming (*www.abh-abnlp.com*). This organization offers lists of certified NLP practitioners in the United States.

ANLP – Association for Neuro Linguistic Programming (*www.anlp.org*). This organization offers a list of certified NLP practitioners in the UK.

ADA – American Diabetes Association (*www.diabetes.org*). This leading charity in the US provides useful resources and information about diabetes.

CNHC – Complementary and Natural Healthcare Council (*www.cnhc.org.uk*). This is the official UK voluntary register of complementary health care practitioners set up by the government and covers complementary health practitioners working in many different categories. If a practitioner has this logo displayed, you may be able to get a referral to them under the NHS, if you ask your GP. (Please be aware: NHS referral choices frequently change and are never guaranteed.)

Diabetes UK – (*www.diabetes.org.uk*). This is a UK diabetes charity that helps to provide support and care for people affected by diabetes. Here you will find the latest news and some helpful resources

GHR – General Hypnotherapy Register (*www.general-hypnotherapy-register.com*). At this register, you'll find a list of practitioners within the field of hypnotherapy and the training of hypnotherapy, so again, do your research.

Low Carb Megastore – (*www.lowcarbmegastore.com*) This is a good online source of mail order online low-carb and sugar-free foods in the UK.

Low Carb Grocery Store - (*http://www.thelowcarbgrocery.com*) This is a good online source of mail order low-carb and sugar-free foods throughout Canada, and the U.S.

Low Carb Connection – (*http://www.locarbconnection.com*) This is a good online source of mail order low-carb and sugar-free foods throughout the U.S.

Dr. Sarah Brewer – (*http://drsarahbrewer.com*) UK doctor Sarah Brewer's website offers excellent information on nutrition and advice and on medical matters generally.

Dr. Mark Hyman – (*http://drhyman.com*). Dr. Hyman is a well-known functional medicine doctor in the US. His website and books offer great information on supporting diets for blood sugar solutions, and all other general medical matters, too.

Sugar Free Megastore – (*www.sugarfreemegastore.com*) – This is another good online source of mail order online low-carb and sugar-free foods in the UK.

NHS 111 – In the UK, dial **111** for non-urgent medical emergencies, when you need medical advice or help but it isn't as serious as an emergency 999 call. This service can dispatch ambulances, if required, but will, in any case, give helpful advice.

Dr. Fox – (*www.doctorfox.co.uk*) Dr. Fox undertakes consultations online for certain prescription medication posted direct to you. UK GMC registered doctors issue the prescriptions. Prescription medicine is supplied from an NHS online pharmacy (delivery within EU). The service is confidential, safe, and fully regulated in the UK.

Any Time Doctor – (*www.anytimedoctor.co.uk*) This site is regulated by The Quality Care Commissions, and all GMC-registered doctors. You can access an online doctor consultation and prescription service.

Online USA Doctors.com – (*http://www.onlineusadoctors.com/*) This site offers telemedicine services offering online doctor consultations, and authoritative medical resources.

Diabetes Education Online – Diabetes Teaching Center online at the University of California, San Francisco (*http://dtc.ucsf.edu*) . This is a very reliable and well-explained resource, if you wish to know any further details about diabetes.

Bibliography

Alberti, K. G. M. M. and P. Zimmet, H. Keen, R. A. Defronzo. *International Textbook of Diabetes Mellitus*, 2nd ed. Chichester, UK: Wiley and Sons Ltd, 1997.

Bandler, R. and J. Grinder. *Trance-formations: Neuro-Linguistic Programming and the Structure of Hypnosis*. Boulder, CO: Real People Press, 1981.

Bartram, Thomas. *Bartram's Encyclopedia of Herbal Medicine*. London: Robinson Publishing, 1998.

Bilous, R., and R. Donnelly. *Handbook of Diabetes 4th ed*. Oxford: Wiley-Blackwell Publishing, 2010.

Brown, P. *The Hypnotic Brain: Hypnotherapy and Social Communication.* New York: Vail-Ballou Press, 1951.

Cefalu, W. T. *Stop Diabetes Now: Controlling Your Disease and Staying Healthy*. London: Penguin Group, 2008.

Chopra, D. *Quantum Healing: Exploring the Frontiers of Mind-Body Medicine.* New York: Bantam Books, 1989.

Cochran, S. V. and F. E. Rabinowitz. *Men and Depression: Clinical and Empirical Perspectives (Practical Resources for the Mental Health Profession)*. San Diego, CA: Academic Press, a division of Elsevier, 2001.

Erickson, M. H. and S. Hershman, I. I. Secter. *The Practical Application of Medical and Dental Hypnosis.* Brunner/Mazel, Inc., 1961.

Erickson, M. H. and E. L. Rossi. *Experiencing Hypnosis: Therapeutic Approaches to Altered States.* New York: Irvington Publishers, 1991.

Hay, Louise. *You Can Heal Your Life*. Carlsbad, CA: Hay House, 1984.

Herbert, N. *Quantum Reality: Beyond the New Physics*. New York: Anchor Books, 1985.

James, T. and L. Flores, J. Schober. (2000) *Hypnosis: A Comprehensive Guide, Producing Deep Trance Phenomena*. New York: Crown House Publishing, 2000.

James, T. and W. Woodsmall. *Time Line Therapy and The Basis of Personality*. Soquel, CA: Meta Publications, 1988.

Kisen. *Yoga Pure and Simple*. London: Ebury Publishing, a division of Penguin Random House, 2001.

McMillan, B. *Atlas of the Human Body*. Ultimo, Australia: Argosy Publishing/Welden Owen, 2008.

Murray, M. T. and J. Pizzorno, L. Pizzorno. *The Encyclopaedia of Healing Foods.* New York: Atria Books, a division of Simon & Schuster, 2005.

Pert, C.B. *Molecules of Emotion: Why You Feel the Way You Feel.* New York: Simon and Schuster, 1997.

Rossi, E. *The Psycho-Biology of Mind-Body Healing.* New York: W. W. Norton and Company, Inc, 1986.

End Notes

1. Chopra, D. *Quantum Healing: Exploring the Frontiers of Mind-Body Medicine*. New York: Bantam Books, 1989. Ch. 3, p. 44. Dr. Chopra explains how Godfrey Raisman, a researcher in Cambridge, proved with an electro microscope that damaged nerve cells can sprout new growth, Ch. 3, p. 47.

2. Dr. Benveniste is a French immunologist famous for his scientific paper alluding to cell memory, published in *Nature,* Vol. 333, 30 June 1988. This scientific paper can be accessed online at *http://www.researchgate.net/publication/20701366_Human_basophil_degranulation_triggered_by_very_dilute_antiserum_against_IgE*. In addition, a good reference is *http://www.sciencedirect.com/science/article/pii/S0007078588800061* to access an article from *The British Homeopathic Journal,* October 1988, Vol. 77, pp. 228-230. abstract, titled 'A turning point for homeopathy'. This is a very good, succinct, and relevant overview of this experiment.

3. *http://www.intropsych.com/ch06_memory/lashleys_research.html*. Gerrig and Zimbardo (2005) Psychology and Life (17th edition: International edition).

4. Talbot, Michael. *The Holographic Universe: The Revolutionary Theory of Reality*. New York: HarperCollins, new edition 1996. *http://www.karlpribram.com* Dr. Tad James, NLP practitioner training, 2011. *https://en.wikipedia.org/wiki/Karl_H._Pribram*

5. Alberti, K. G. M. M. and P. Zimmet, H. Keen, R. A. Defronzo. *International Textbook of Diabetes Mellitus*, 2nd ed. Chichester, UK: Wiley and Sons Ltd, 1997. Ch.18, 'The hypothalamus, neuropeptides and diabetes', p. 396.
   Rossi. E. *The Psycho-Biology of Mind-Body Healing*. New York: W. W.Norton and Company, Inc, 1986, Ch. 8, 'Mind modulation of the endocrine system', p. 189, Table 4, 'The multiple functions of some hormones that have related functions in mind and body'.
   Pert, C.B. *Molecules of Emotion: Why You Feel the Way You Feel*. New York: Simon and Schuster, 1997, Ch. 3, 'Peptide Generation: A Continued Lecture', p. 66.

6. Evidence for the link between colds and emotion. The following articles can be found by searching pubmed.gov and typing in the relevant PMID number listed:
   Epidemiology. 2001 May;12(3):345-9. 'A cohort study of stress and the common cold'. Takkouche B, Regueira C, Gestal-Otero JJ. PMID: 11338315.
   Health Psychol. 1998 May;17(3):214-23. 'Types of stressors that increase susceptibility to the common cold in healthy adults'. Cohen S, Frank E, Doyle WJ, Skoner DP, Rabin BS, Gwaltney JM Jr. PMID: 9619470.
   J Psychosom Res. 2001 Jan;50(1):21-7. 'Psychological job demands as a risk factor for common cold in a Dutch working population'. Mohren DC, Swaen GM, Borm PJ, Bast A, Galama JM. PMID: 11259797.

Behav Med. 1992 Fall;18(3):115-20. 'Development of common cold symptoms following experimental rhinovirus infection is related to prior stressful life events'. Stone AA, Bovbjerg DH, Neale JM, Napoli A, Valdimarsdottir H, Cox D, Hayden FG, Gwaltney JM Jr. PMID: 1330102.

7. Chopra, D. *Quantum Healing: Exploring the Frontiers of Mind-Body Medicine.* New York: Bantam Books, 1989. Ch. 8, 'Silent Witness', p. 133.

8. Professor Guru Aithal, Nottingham University Hospitals Trust.

9. Medical definitions and referencing of hormones. Diabetes Teaching Center at the University of California, San Francisco, *http://dtc.ucsf.edu* .

10. Murray, M. T. and J. Pizzorno, L. Pizzorno. *The Encyclopaedia of Healing Foods.* New York: Atria Books, a division of Simon & Schuster, 2005, Ch. 4, 'Food Prescriptions for Specific Diseases', p. 765.

11. *http://examine.com/supplements/vitex-agnus-castus/*
    http://www.webmd.com/vitamins-supplements/ingredientmono-968-chasteberry.aspx?active ingredientid=968&activeingredientname=chasteberry

12. Visualization Case 1971 by Dr. O. Carl Simonton, a radiologist at the University of Texas.
    http://www.thesimontondocumentary.org/about_dr_simonton

13. Norman Cousins. *Head First: The Biology of Hope.* New York: Dutton, 1989.

14. 'Reversal of type 2 diabetes: normalization of beta cell function in association with decreased pancreas and liver triacylglycerol' (Lim EL, Hollingsworth KG, Aribisala BS, Chen MJ, Mathers JC, Taylor R., 2011). This study was published in *Diabetologia*, a journal of clinical and experimental research within the field of diabetes (2011 Oct;54(10):2506-14. doi: 10.1007/s00125-011-2204-7. Epub 2011 Jun 9; *www.diabetologia-journal.org*).

15. A 2005 study that took place in the Department of Psychiatry at the Medical School of Ohio – 'Biofeedback-assisted relaxation in type 2 diabetes' (McGinnis RA, McGrady A, Cox SA, Grower-Dowling KA, 2005). Published in the journal *Diabetes Care* (2005 Sep;28(9):2145-9).

16. Joseph E. Pizzorno and Michael T. Murray, *The Encyclopaedia of Natural Medicine* (Little Brown, 1999), Ch. 15, p. 479.

17. 'From mental power to muscle power: gaining strength by using the mind', Ranganathan VK[1], Siemionow V, Liu JZ, Sahgal V, Yue GH, Department of Biomedical Engineering/ND20, The Lerner Research Institute, The Cleveland Clinic Foundation, 9500 Euclid Avenue, Cleveland, OH 44195, USA, 2004. *http://www.ncbi.nlm.nih.gov/pubmed/14998709*

18. The University of Toronto, Centre for Sleep and Chronobiology. Dr. Harvey Moldofsky et al., *Psychosom Med* 1975;37:341-51.

19. 'The effect of a multivitamin and mineral supplement on infection and quality of life' (Thomas A. Barringer, MD; Julienne K. Kirk, PharmD; Amy C. Santaniello, PharmD; Kristie Long Foley, PhD; and Robert Michielutte, PhD; 2003). *http://annals.org/article. aspx?articleid=716096*

20. Cefalu, William T, MD and Hu, Frank B. MD, PhD, Louisiana State University *http://care.diabetesjournals.org/content/27/11/2741.long* (doi: 10.2337/diacare.27.11.2741 *Diabetes Care,* November 2004, vol. 27, no. 11 2741-2751).

21. 'Antidiabetic activity of aloe vera juice. Clinical trial in new cases of diabetes mellitus', Yong-chaiyudha S, Rungpitarangsi V, Bunyapraphatsara N, Chokechaijaroenporn O, Department of Preventive and Social Medicine, Faculty of Medicine Siriraj Hospital, Mahidol University, 1996. *http://www.ncbi.nlm.nih.gov/pubmed/23195077*

22. James, T. and L. Flores, J. Schober. *Hypnosis: A Comprehensive Guide, Producing Deep Trance Phenomena*. New York: Crown House Publishing, 2000, Ch.1, 'Introduction: The Mind/Body Connection', p. 5.

23. 'Optical differences in cases of multiple personality disorder', Miller SD, 1989, *http://www.ncbi.nlm.nih.gov/pubmed/2760599*

24. For an extensive list of sugar alcohols and a good practical example of working out the true carbohydrate amount, you can visit *http://dtc.ucsf.edu/living-with-diabetes/diet-and-nutrition/understanding-carbohydrates/counting-carbohydrates/learning-to-read-labels/counting-sugar-alcohols/*

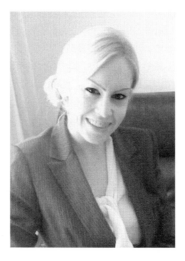

About the Author
Dr. Emma Mardlin

As a trained psychotherapist and holding a PhD in Mind Body Medicine, Dr Emma Mardlin works with both adults and children in clinical practice; working with the human psychology, unconscious mind, and entire neurology to activate positive results in terms of health, well-being, and professional performance. Emma is co-founder and partner to The Pinnacle Practice, a health and well-being clinic and training consultancy in Nottingham and London. Alongside this, Emma and her partner also operate a privately funded charity division of their business for individuals in severe need, as well as taking UK NHS referrals when the system permits.

At The Pinnacle Practice Emma sees individuals with a host of life challenges from psychological and physical health concerns and conditions, to severe traumas, and people in need of general life support, personal and professional development, or understanding oneself to get the very best results in life.

Emma further trains and lectures public organizations, government departments, and private companies in the UK and The United Arab Emirates; writing and delivering requested courses in all aspects of stress management, communication, leadership, presenting, and utilizing the mind for maximum positive results in health, education, and business. Emma also provides professional practitioner qualifications in Clinical Hypnotherapy and Neuro Linguistic Programming. She also writes professionally for numerous journals and media.

As a dedicated individual, Emma displays a genuine passion and energy for all she does, integrating her vast personal and professional life experiences to help others.

For additional resources and information you can visit:

www.dr-em.co.uk
www.pinnacleminds.co.uk
em_mardlin@twitter.com

PROGRESS NOTES

Where am I now?

Where do I really want to be?

_____

_____

_____

_____

_____

_____

_____

_____

_____

_____

_____

_____

_____

_____

_____

What changes am I now going to apply?

FINDHORN PRESS

Life-Changing Books

Consult our catalogue online
(with secure order facility) on
www.findhornpress.com

For information on the Findhorn Foundation:
www.findhorn.org